Aromatherapy for Travellers

About the Author

Jude Brown practises aromatherapy in London. She plays an active role with the Give To The Earth Foundation, a charitable organization which supports social and environmental activities across the globe.

Aromatherapy for Travellers

HOW TO USE ESSENTIAL OILS FOR HEALTH AND
WELL-BEING WHILE TRAVELLING

Jude Brown

Thorsons
An Imprint of HarperCollins*Publishers*

Thorsons
An Imprint of HarperCollinsPublishers
77–85 Fulham Palace Road,
Hammersmith, London W6 8JB
1160 Battery Sreet
San Francisco, California 94111–1213

Published by Thorsons 1995
3 5 7 9 10 8 6 4 2

A catalogue record for this book
is available from the British Library

ISBN 0 7225 3120 6

Printed and bound in Great Britain by
Caledonian International Book Manufacturing Ltd, Glasgow

Contents

Aromatherapy is a form of complementary medicine. Consult your doctor if you have any doubt concerning your state of health prior to or during travelling, especially if you are taking medication. The author and the publishers disclaim any responsibility for any adverse reaction caused by inappropriate use of essential oils and/or use of poor quality products.

Acknowledgements

The author would like to thank the following:
Ziva Belic, International Aromatherapy School, London
and Abu Dhabi; Audrey Barned, Hummingbird Haven,
Ocho Rios; Ellen Liberatori, Give to the Earth Foundation
c/o Aveda Minneapolis; M. Serpico, University College
London; Dr. D. Spengler, Psychoneuro Immunology
Research Centre, Weisbaden; also Terry Beaumont, Ita
O'Brien, Pam Colbourne, Joseph Houseal, Tim Maxwell,
Pella Munday, Philip Rushton and Tony Troy; and Christine
Wildwood for her valuable input.

Introduction

The bounty of good health is the greatest of all gifts.
—'Abdu'l–Baha

Whether you are travelling for business or pleasure, using aromatherapy can help you make the most of the experience. Although travel is often exciting, it can also be tiring and stressful. Essential oils are invaluable for the traveller, as they can help treat a wide variety of ailments, both physical and mental. This book provides you with advice on using aroma-therapy while you are away from home – all in an easy-to-carry format ideal for the traveller.

Travelling is big business. The travel industry is currently rated as the world's largest and fastest-growing industry, accounting for £1 trillion (quin-tillion) of expenditure worldwide. According to the World Tourism Organisation Annual Report (1993), in 1992, UK residents alone spent £25 billion on an estimated 30 million trips abroad; £9.2 billion was spent on business trips, while £11.2 billion account-ed for leisure vacations (the rest of the expenditure was not specified by the report). An estimated 50 million people will be travelling by air every year over the next decade. That is a lot of movement.

Although we are now accustomed to travel, we

can still run into problems while on the move. During the journey we may face travel sickness or backache; and once we reach our destination, we expose ourselves to unfamiliar foods, water, weather conditions and bugs. The best we can do is protect and prepare ourselves for any eventuality, and we can do that with the help of aromatherapy.

In common with other natural remedies, aromatherapy is becoming increasingly popular. A successful trend has recently emerged in the travel industry where airlines, becoming more aware of 'eco-nomic' practices, have started to provide aromatherapy and similar health-orientated services to customers. Virgin Atlantic offers 'Aromamassage' to business travellers and has opened the first pre-flight treatment centre at London's Heathrow Airport; Air New Zealand sells a 'Revival on Arrival' aromatherapy mini-kit through its in-flight magazine; and in 1994, Japan Air became the latest airline to introduce a form of massage on flights. Available only to passengers travelling first-class, this upper-body treatment is based on acupressure. These wonderful ideas can ease the strain of air travel, but aromatherapy can offer the traveller so much more.

In my research for this book, I have discovered that there are many different types of traveller, and that all have particular needs. The guidelines contained in this book are relevant to everyone who travels. If you are a business traveller, aromatherapy can alleviate the effects of jet-lag so that, despite a long-haul flight which can deplete your energy, you can face that important meeting alert, refreshed and ready to do business. If you are a backpacker, aromatherapy ensures that your surroundings – whether they are unfamiliar hostels or campsites which have played host to plenty before you – are purified and aesthetically pleasant. For the family taking an annual holiday, aromatherapy can make travel sickness and anxiety a thing of the past. And insect-repellent formulas made from essential oils can be put to good use by every traveller.

Whatever your needs, this book will enable you to make the most of aromatherapy while on your travels. It gives you background to the art of aromatherapy, introduces you to the essential oils and carrier oils that should be in your 'travel kit' and provides an A-Z guide to common ailments which can mar a travel experience. There is even a quick reference chart for use in an emergency.

Although an ancient practice, aromatherapy has a significant role to play in this modern, high-tech age. As travel features increasingly in our lives, we can benefit from the use of essential oils while on the move. The formulas in the following pages are not just a pleasure to use but they work too; I have used them on myself and on many willing participants encountered on my travels. Once you have mastered the art of aromatherapy you will have opened the door to a invaluable lifelong adventure in itself.

CHAPTER ONE

What is Aromatherapy?

The History of Aromatherapy

Aromatherapy has a long history. Herbs and aromatic oils have been used therapeutically by many different civilizations for thousands of years. The use of plant-derived medicines to treat and prevent ailments is thought to have originated in India and China. The practice was extremely popular with the Chinese emperors. Kwang-ti (450 BC) was the first to document the medicinal use of roots, barks and fruit such as opium and pomegranate. Shen Nung, who lived sometime between 1000 and 700 BC, spent most of his time compiling the *Pen Tsao* (Great Herbal), a comprehensive glossary of herbs, preparations and remedies. Egyptian priests, who also fulfilled the roles of doctor and embalmer, used aromatic concoctions in religious ceremonies and for medicinal purposes. Seven sacred oils have been found at burial sites of pharaohs, which are thought to have been intended for use in religious rites. Although the exact reason for their use is currently being researched, the contents of excavated small, alabaster vessels have been identified as aromatic resin, most of which was made from frankincense, myrrh and olibanum.

Scrolls such as the Ebers Papyrus (1550 BC), which came to light during 19th-century excavations, document the use of up to 800 herbal remedies. Included in this medical compendium are remedies for the treatment of lice and fleas. Alexandria, the destroyed Egyptian city which played host to the greatest library of the ancient world, was an education centre for the Greeks and, later, for Roman physicians. It was also, from 300 BC to AD 100, the perfume centre of the world. Among Alexander the Great's spoils of war were herbs and medicinal references from as far away as Tibet.

The Greek physicians were widely respected – and employed by the Romans – for their medicinal knowledge. Hippocrates, physician and philosopher (460–377 BC), was called the 'Father of Medicine' due to his work *Corpus Hippocratus*, a standard textbook of its day on the treatment of the body with the help of plants and diet. Other notables were Dioscorides, a surgeon in Nero's army, whose *Materia Medica* remained a classic textbook until the Renaissance, and Galen (AD 131–201), the inventor of the cold cream, a formula still used in the cosmetics industry today. This creation came about while Galen was physician to the Roman gladiators. He saw a need for a viscous substance to carry the resins and herbs he used to treat the wounds of the fighters.

During the period known in Europe as the 'Dark Ages', the Arab civilization continued to advance medical and scientific research. The Arabians perfected the method of extracting essences called distillation, which is the most common form of extraction used today. Yakuso Al-Kindi (AD 850) wrote the first book on the subject, *Book of Perfumes and Distillation*. Avicenna (AD 980–1037), a chemist, physician and philosopher, became the first person to distil essence of rose, known as rose attar. This is still an extremely expensive process as it requires vast amounts of rose petals (a by-product of this process is rose-water). Known as the 'Prince of Medicine' in the Arab world, Avicenna compiled *The Qanun* (The Canon of Medicine) which, until the 16th century, was the definitive source of reference for distillation and medicine. The 'perfumes of Arabia' were brought to Europe by knights returning from the Crusades and the Arab Moors who established citadels in southern Spain. By the 12th century, essential-oil producers, distilleries and apothecary guilds were well established.

Throughout the plagues that swept across Europe, the distillers who extracted the essences from herbs and flowers were the only people immune to the deadly disease. People resorted to carrying aromatic flowers and plants with them and burning incense made from pine, cedar and cypress to dispel disease and the offending odour that accompanied those affected by it. During the Great Plague (1665–6), the now popular nursery rhyme 'Ring a ring a roses' was coined as more people looked to aromatic flowers and herbs to heal themselves. Nicholas Culpeper's *Complete Herbal and English Physician* documented the use of herbs and flowers for medicinal and culinary purposes and was used as a reference by those treating the Plague. It is still in print today.

The discovery of the Americas introduced new plants, such as wintergreen, to Europe and many were transported to botanical gardens for research, as found at Kew Gardens in England. The Spanish conquistadors gathered resources from Montezuma's botanical gardens and learnt of healing herbs used by Aztec physicians. The Inca practice of chewing cocoa leaves also became widely used by the Spaniards.

During the first world war (1914–18), French doctors burnt bushes of lavender and rosemary in hospital wards to prevent the spread of infection. French scientist, René Maurice Gattefossé, coined the term 'aromatherapy' and pioneered modern scientific research into the properties of essential oils. While conducting experiments into their cosmetic uses, he burnt his hand quite severely and plunged it into a vat of lavender oil. The burn healed remarkably quickly, leading him to expand his research into the healing properties of the oils. Marguerite Maury, a biochemist who worked with Gattefossé, was the pioneer of aromatherapy massage treatment.

The Power of Essential Oils

The term 'aromatherapy' refers to the use of essential oils to aid the healing process and restore equilibrium to the body. Essential oils are powerful substances extracted from odoriferous herbs, flowers, barks and fruits, mainly via a distillation process which harnesses the 'heart' of the plant – its chemical components. The most odoriferous plants are found in the tropics where there is an abundance of solar energy. Essential oils are stored as microdroplets in the glands of the plant. They disperse through the walls of the glands, circulate throughout the plant and eventually spread over the surface before evaporating into the atmosphere, filling the air with fragrance.

Essential oils have come to be known as the 'hormones' of the plant, but scientists are still trying to pinpoint their role. Some maintain that these essences help the natural selection process by attracting or repelling insects, as well as protecting the root of the plant against parasites. Others suggest that essential oils are a by-product of the photosynthesis process. Essential oils, in fact, are not 'oily' substances – if dropped onto blotting paper, the oil will leave no trace once it has evaporated.

When used sensibly, essential oils can stimulate the functions of our bodies with no adverse side-effects. This is due to the remarkable fact that the DNA patterns of plants and humans differ only slightly. The most compelling aspect of essential oils is their ability to penetrate the skin and tone circulatory systems. Once excreted, they leave behind only minute traces, unlike manufactured petrochemical drugs. When topically applied they can improve the condition of the skin, restore tone and elasticity and alleviate imbalances such as acne or eczema. They can even heal wounds, leaving little or no scarring. Today, French doctors prescribe aromatherapy treatments alongside 'traditional' medicine.

Essential oils are quite remarkable, a testament to the powerful allies with which nature has provided us to maintain health and wellbeing. They are generally antiseptic, antibacterial and regenerative, and each essence has numerous therapeutic uses. They have the added bonus of being completely harmless to the environment.

Apart from the physical benefits of essential oils, they also have the ability to affect our moods by stimulating the olfactory nerves in the brain. Modern science has determined that there is a relationship between what we smell, how we feel and what we perceive. A familiar, reassuring smell is 'familiar' only because our brain has registered that smell at some time in the past and associated it with a place or person we hold dear in memory. For the traveller, a fragrance may stimulate the impression of colour, taste, sound and feel of the visited region or country. When essential oils are inhaled, they can have a powerful effect, making you feel relaxed or alert. Some essential oils have a dual effect on the mind and the body depending upon the dosage and method used. A typical example is lavender, which in small dosages in an aromatic bath is quite relaxing but can be stimulating if the dosage is increased. Regular use of essential oils can help you build a resistance to infection and strengthen your immune system.

Essential oils have a shelf life of around a year, although some retain their properties for much longer and mature like a good wine when unopened. Distilled from petals, herbs, roots and barks, they are packaged in tinted bottles for protection from ultraviolet light which can dissipate the chemicals. Up to a tonne of rose petals is required to distil 1 kilogram of rose attar, which is why this oil is quite expensive.

Aromatherapists blend essential oils taking into account the volatility of the oil, which relates to the rate of evaporation and the effect the essence will have on the body. This effect is determined by the chemical constituents, which are compositions of alcohols, acids, terpenes and ketones acting in synergy.

In aromatherapy, a musical analogy is often used to describe the fragrance of essential oils. Depending on its qualities, an oil is described as a top, middle or base 'note':

- Top notes – perceived immediately; fast-acting; the quickest to evaporate; the most refreshing and uplifting to the mind and body.
- Middle notes – moderately fast-acting; dense odour; stimulating to bodily functions such as digestion, excretion and menstruation.
- Base notes – slowest to evaporate; most persistent and calming odour.

Visiting an Aromatherapist

Treat yourself to a visit to a professional aromatherapist. You should choose the practitioner carefully, either on a friend's recommendation or through a professional body such as the IFA (International Federation Of Aromatherapists) or IPTI (Independent Professional Therapists International) who can supply a list of practitioners in your area (for addresses of these organizations, see *Appendix 4, Professional Associations*). When you ring to arrange an appointment, do not be afraid to ask questions: some practitioners specialize in certain types of treatment, such as beauty therapy, which may or may not be what you are looking for.

Conscientious aromatherapists take into account your physical, emotional and mental state before choosing and blending the oils and commencing the treatment. This is because aromatherapy is a 'whole-person' therapy, and can have powerful effects on the mind as well as the body.

Essential oils can be used in a variety of ways (*see pages* 12–16), but the most popular method with aromatherapists is massage. After a relaxing 'aromamassage', refrain from taking a shower or bath for at least six hours. This allows the essential oils to be assimilated throughout your body and tone your whole system before being excreted through the skin (perspiration), through exhaling or through primary excretory functions (urine and faeces).

I find it beneficial to have a couple of professional aromatherapy treatments a month or so before travelling to help build up a resistance to infection.

Buying Essential Oils

Before buying essential oils, make sure you fully understand how to use the oils effectively and safely. An aromatherapist would be more than happy to take the time to explain this to you, and would rather you ask than misuse the oils.

You can buy essential oils from an aromatherapist, a health-food shop or a reputable herbal retailer. For a list of retailers and suppliers, *see page* 152. Always examine the label carefully. Essential oils should be labelled '100 per cent pure'. Do not buy oils labelled 'nature identical', as these are manufactured, not organic, perfumes unsuitable for therapuetic purposes. In time and with practice, your nose will be the best form of 'quality control' available to you.

Base Oils

Essential oils are generally too powerful to use directly on the skin and must be diluted in a base or 'carrier' oil. These cold-pressed oils are derived from nuts and seeds and are beneficial in their own right. Packed with vitamins, minerals and proteins, they have an affinity with the skin and can penetrate and nourish its surface. When applying essential oils to the skin, such as in an aromatherapy massage, the base oil will 'carry' the essence and ensure an effective treatment. To use essential oils in the bath, dilute a few drops in half a teaspoon (2.5 ml) of base oil first to ensure that the essential oils do not evaporate too quickly and that the aroma is lingering and released slowly.

Baby oil and other synthetic oils are not suitable for aromatherapy. They have large molecules that do not allow for penetration or nourishment of the skin's surface. They do nothing more than sit on the surface of the skin and can even block pores. Appropriate base oils, such as the types described below, can be bought from health-food shops or from any of the outlets listed on page 152. Cold-pressed base oils have a shelf life of two to three years.

Almond Oil
Source: nut
SUITABLE FOR: ALL SKIN TYPES

A pale-yellow oil with a light consistency. Ideal for removing eye make-up and nourishing the eye area. (Apply a small amount with the fingertips, dotting around the eye, then leave for a minute or two. Blot the excess with a tissue.) Can be used on its own as a base oil.

Apricot Kernel Oil
Source: nut
SUITABLE FOR: ALL SKIN TYPES, ESPECIALLY DRY AND SENSITIVE

A pale-yellow oil with a slightly rich consistency. Relieves itching, dryness and inflammation. Can be used on its own as a base oil.

Sesame Seed Oil
Source: seed
SUITABLE FOR: ALL SKIN TYPES

A dark-yellow oil with a rich consistency. Contains a small amount of a natural sun filter and protects against UVA/UVB rays (to the equivalent of about factor 2). Soothes inflamed skin and eradicates scars. Suitable for use in a blend of base oils, comprising about 5 per cent.

Wheatgerm Oil
Source: *seed*
SUITABLE FOR: ALL SKIN TYPES

A dark-yellow oil, rich in Vitamin E, wheatgerm is excellent for keeping crow's-feet at bay. Good for preserving blends of essential oils. Oxygenates skin and repairs damage. Suitable for use in a blend of base oils, comprising about 5 per cent.

Travel Blend
For your travels, the following blends of base oils are suitably versatile. Choose the right one for your skin type.

OILY/NORMAL SKIN
- 90% almond oil
- 5% sesame oil
- 5% wheatgerm oil

DRY/SENSITIVE SKIN
- 90% apricot kernel oil
- 5% sesame oil
- 5% wheatgerm oil

Using Essential Oils

Now that you have an idea of how to blend your oils, let us look at the ways in which essential oils can be used.

Aromamassage

Massage is a valuable lifetime skill which stimulates blood flow and eases muscular pain. To massage ourselves or others the basic rules are easy to follow. When working on the legs, thighs, arms, neck or chest, always massage towards the heart. For the stomach, work in a clockwise direction. Massage the lower back in an up-and-outwards direction. Always maintain contact between the hand and the area being treated, making one stroke after another in the same direction.

For facial massage concentrate on small, circular movements, particularly around the sinuses, temples and forehead. Use a base oil, but no essential oils, around the eye area. After bathing, use 2–4 teaspoons of base oil mixed with your favourite blend of essential oils for an aromatic body rub to condition skin and increase suppleness.

DOSAGE

One drop of essential oil to 5 ml of base oil.

In the Bath

An aromatic bath is a wonderful, relaxing experience which allows essential oils to treat the whole body. Run a bath. Mix the essential oil with the base oil and add the mixture to the water, making sure it is well dispersed. Enjoy a good soak, for at least 10 minutes, and be sure to secure doors and windows to prevent vapours from escaping.

Adding base oil to the water prevents the essential

oils from evaporating too quickly; the base oil nourishes the skin and, over a period of time, your skin
texture will improve immensely.

DOSAGE

Maximum of six drops of essential oil suspended in
2.5 ml of base oil.

Compress

Hot and cold compresses are useful in reducing
pain, inflammation and body temperature. Compresses are pieces of cloth or gauze soaked in a
solution of water (preferably distilled) and essential
oil. The size of cloth needed depends on the area
being treated. For example, use a handkerchief to
treat the forehead and a flannel or small towel for
the stomach or sprains. Excess solution should be
squeezed from the saturated cloth before the compress is applied to the affected area.

DOSAGE

Maxiumum of three drops of essential oil to 2 litres
of water.

Foot Soak

Soaking your aching feet in a bowl of aromatic hot
water is a soothing experience. It is also great for
combating foot odour. Soak feet for 15 minutes,
topping up with hot water when necessary. Make
sure that the water is not too hot.

DOSAGE

Maximum of two drops of essential oil to 2 litres of water.

Shower

After washing, enjoy an aromatic finishing rinse by adding essential oils to your loofah, sponge or wash-cloth and briskly rub your body while standing beneath the shower. This action stimulates circulation while providing an aromatic bacteria protector. Breathe in the essential vapours.

DOSAGE

Maximum of three drops of essential oil.

Tissue / Handkerchief

To inhale essential oils quickly and efficiently, add to a tissue or handkerchief and sniff when required.

DOSAGE

One drop of essential oil per tissue or handkerchief.

Vapour Ring

The vapour ring is an ingenious modern invention which can be bought from health-food shops or aromatherapy suppliers. The porcelain or ceramic rings are designed to fit snugly on a light bulb; the essences are added to the groove and the heat from the bulb warms the contents, thereby dispersing the molecules into the atmosphere.

DOSAGE

Maximum of eight drops of essential oil to a little
water.

CHAPTER TWO

The Essential Travel Kit

Before you travel, you will need to put together an aromatherapy kit. This does not have to take up much luggage space as a small, neat box will hold everything you need to treat most of the minor physical and mental ailments you may encounter on your travels.

What Will I Need?

Your essential travel kit should contain the following:

- *Eight essential oils: chamomile, eucalyptus, geranium, lavender, lemongrass, peppermint, rosemary and tea tree (see page 20).*
- *200 ml (7 fl oz) of base oil (sufficient for a two-to-three week trip).*
- *10 ml (2 teaspoons) of almond oil or vitamin E oil to be used sparingly on the brow and under the eye to nourish this delicate area.*

- Three empty plastic bottles (preferably recycled and with spray attachments). One should have a capacity of 100 ml (10 tablespoons) and the other two should be able to hold 50 ml (10 teaspoons) of fluid. These should be available from your local herbalist or health-food shop, or see Appendix 3, Retailers and Suppliers.
- One vapour ring.
- One pack of chamomile tea bags (optional).
- Rosewater (optional for extremely dry/sensitive skins).
- Gauze (available from pharmacies).
- 1 flannel or washcloth.

Measurements

It is important to measure precisely the amount of essential oil and base oil you use in any preparation. Before you set off, you need to be sure that you have a foolproof system of measurement that you can use on your travels. This does not have to be complicated.

In this book, essential oils are measured in drops. Most bottles of essential oil have built-in pipettes which allow you to dispense one drop at a time. If this is not the case, buy a pipette for each bottle to add to your travel kit. The base oils, which are used for diluting the essential oils, are measured in millilitres (ml). The maxiumum amount you will need to use at any time is 20 ml, which is sufficient for one to two body applications. Translating millilitre measurements into spoon measurements can make life easier, as you can add a set of measuring spoons to your travel kit. It is much simpler, however, to use the cap of the base oil bottle. As bottle caps vary in depth, work out before you leave how many capfuls equal the measurements given in the box below, and make a note. Larger measurements are sometimes given for water. To measure this out, use an empty water bottle.

2.5 ml = ½ *teaspoon*
5 ml = 1 *teaspoon*
10 ml = 1 *tablespoon*
20 ml = 2 *tablespoons*

Preparation and Safety

Once you have purchased your oils, experiment with them at home or prepare formulas you are most likely to need (depending on your destination). Shake the mixture well and store in a dark place at least a week before your travels. This allows the oils to fuse, resulting in a more full-bodied aroma. Some companies provide ready-mixed essences suitable for travel (*see Retailers and Suppliers, page* 152).

It is also easier to transport essential oils once they have been diluted in base oil. As they are live, organic substances, essential oils tend to expand when in a pressurized environment such as an air cabin, and the base oil gives them room to do so safely within the container. Keep oils away from heat sources and/or bright lights as these influences can impair quality and effectiveness. Likewise, make sure they are well out of the reach of children.

The Traveller's Eight Essential Oils

Chamomile
Herb
PARTS USED: FLOWER AND LEAVES

HABITAT: ENGLAND, FRANCE, HUNGARY, ASIA, SOUTH AMERICA

Chamomile is one of the most popular and well-known herbs. Used for medicinal and culinary purposes throughout the ages, this delicately fragrant plant was grown in abundance for its refreshing, therapeutic tea. In Elizabethan England it earned the reputation of being the 'plant's physician', as when it was planted next to sickly plants, their condition would improve.

Chamomile essential oil contains an aromatic substance called azulene to which its anti-inflammatory and regenerative properties are mostly attributed. This chemical is not detectable in the plant, but is developed during the distillation process. Even in its raw state, however, chamomile is beneficial. Chamomile tea bags placed on tired eyes are excellent at reducing swelling and irritation.

PROPERTIES
analgesic
anti-inflammatory
diuretic
skin rejuvenating
sedative

USE FOR
burns
diarrhoea
depression
eczema
fever
hayfever
insomnia
nausea
nerves
sprains
sunburn

Eucalyptus
Tree

PARTS USED: LEAVES AND TWIGS

HABITAT: AUSTRALIA/TASMANIA, INDIA, SOUTHERN
EUROPE, SOUTHERN AFRICA, TAHITI, USA

The eucalyptus tree is indigenous to Australia and
Tasmania. During the 19th century its significance
as a therapeutic agent grew rapidly and production
spread to the above areas due to the wonderful properties in the leaves. The active ingredient, eucalyptol,
is present in only minute quantities, so vast amounts

of leaves are required to extract the essence – 1 tonne for 1 litre of essential oil.

PROPERTIES
analgesic
antibiotic
antiseptic
antiviral
decongestant
deodorizing
insect-repellent

USE FOR
Candida albicans
cystitis
fever
muscular strain
sore throat
sunburn
upset stomach

Geranium
Flowering plant
PARTS USED: FLOWERS, LEAVES AND STALKS

HABITAT: ALGERIA, CHINA, EGYPT, FRANCE, MADAGASCAR, MOROCCO, USA

Geranium flourishes in low ground and is fast becoming recognized as a plant of various uses. In late spring, the plant produces flowers ranging in colour from pale pink to purple. Geranium essential oil balances the nervous system and eases menstrual pain. A potent antiseptic, it is indispensable for general use. The scent is delightfully refreshing and, like all perennials used for producing essential oil, tonnes of flowers, leaves and stalks are required to obtain the oil, which is a light yellow-green.

PROPERTIES
antiseptic
astringent
sedative

USE FOR
anxiety
chilblains
diarrhoea
frostbite
menstrual pain
pre-menstrual syndrome
nerves
sunburn
throat problems

Lavender
Shrub
PARTS USED: FLOWERING BUDS

HABITAT: AUSTRALIA/TASMANIA, ENGLAND, FRANCE, SCANDINAVIA, SCOTLAND, USA

Lavender is a much-respected herb. Although indigenous to mountain regions, it is hardy enough to grow just about anywhere. The essential oil is widely used in the perfume and food industries. The

Greeks held the plant in such high esteem that they named a Syrian city Nardus, after *narda*, the Greek for lavender. The chief constituents which make lavender essential oil so valuable are linalool and linalyl acetate, to which lavender owes its charming fragrance.

PROPERTIES
antibiotic
antiseptic
antiviral
sedative
stimulating (immune system)

USE FOR
acne
burns
cuts
depression
headaches
inflammation
influenza
insomnia
nausea
nervous tension
scarring
sunburn

Lemongrass
Grass
PARTS USED: ALL

HABITAT: AFRICA, BRAZIL, INDIA, SRI LANKA, SEYCHELLES, WEST INDIES

This species of grass is cultivated in vast quantities purely for its essential oil, which is the main component for many successful contemporary fragrances. In the past, the grass was used to produce a tea reputed to ward off fevers, hence its nickname 'fever grass'.

The pungent, refreshing, citrus-like smell is due to the vast quantities of the chemical citrol present in the grass. The plant is grown in subtropical and tropical climates for a good reason: insects find citrol repellent, and many homes in the West Indies have lemongrass planted around the perimeter to ward off bugs.

PROPERTIES
disinfectant
general tonic
insect-repellent

USE FOR
fevers
headaches
infections
sore throats

Peppermint
Herb
PARTS USED: ALL

HABITAT: CANADA, CHINA, EUROPE, JAPAN, USA

Peppermint has been used for centuries as a flavouring and medicinal agent. Its congenial, uplifting fragrance probably accounts for why the Greeks and Romans were particularly partial to this herb. Pliny (23–79 AD), the Roman historian and philosopher, recalls how the Greeks would crown themselves with peppermint garlands during ceremonial events. The Romans would infuse vast amounts of peppermint in water, and add the liquid to their waterfalls to purify and uplift their surroundings. The USA is now the most important producer of peppermint essential oil worldwide; in Michigan, thousands of acres of land are planted with nothing but peppermint.

The chief component of this volatile oil is menthol which has a powerful analgesic and antispasmodic effect on the body, making the essence an excellent painkiller.

PROPERTIES
anti-inflammatory
antiseptic
decongestant
insect-repellent
reduces body temperature

USE FOR

bad breath
catarrh
fatigue
flatulence
headaches
indigestion
influenza
poor circulation
migraines
nausea
nervous disorders
seasickness
upset stomach

Rosemary
Herb

PARTS USED: FLOWERS AND LEAVES

HABITAT: FRANCE, ITALY, SPAIN, JAPAN

Ancient civilizations were familiar with rosemary's ability to improve the memory, and for this reason the herb became the symbol of fidelity between lovers. During the middle ages it was used in Europe for religious ceremonies; a rosemary bush was presented to wedding guests as a symbol of luck and fidelity.

Rosemary essential oil has powerful tonic properties which are best utilized for backache and muscular problems. It is a powerful stimulant and excellent for encouraging healthy hair growth and preventing hair loss.

PROPERTIES
physical and mental stimulant

USE FOR
acne
arthritis
coughs
dandruff
depression
fatigue
headaches
influenza
migraine
muscular conditions

Tea Tree
Tree

PARTS USED: LEAVES AND TWIGS

HABITAT: AUSTRALIA/TASMANIA

This medicinal tree has increased in popularity since the mid-1970s. The tea tree is indigenous to Australia but research is currently being conducted to see how it adapts to the habitat of the western USA. The Aborigines have used the leaves for centuries to treat all sorts of ailments, but the name was coined by sailors voyaging with Captain Cook who, missing their daily cuppa, boiled the leaves to produce a 'tea' which retained its curative properties.

Scientific research into this remarkable oil conducted after the first world war validated its healing attributes. It was supplied as a healing aid to the

Australian Army during the second world war. Research resumed in the 1970s and is still going on to identify the remarkable components of this essential oil which is 100 times more potent than carbolic acid, yet safe for use on most skins.

PROPERTIES
antibacterial
antifungal
antiviral

USE FOR
burns
Candida albicans
cystitis
inflammation
rashes
shock
sunburn

CHAPTER THREE

A-Z of Ailments and Aromatherapy Treatments

Aches

Whether you are travelling by air, road or rail, sitting for hours during a long journey can tax your nerves and leave your body depleted of energy and worse for wear. Painful knees, cramp, lower-back pain and finding yourself with little room to stretch your legs do not make for a comfortable experience.

With the help of aromatherapy you can do much to prepare your body for the trip or alleviate discomfort. Before setting off, relax in an aromatic bath to prime your body (and your nerves!) for the journey ahead. Add the following formula to your bath water, making sure it is well dispersed:

> 2 drops lavender oil
> 3 drops rosemary oil
> 2.5 ml base oil

To loosen muscles and encourage circulation, prepare the following aromatic after-bath rub:

2 drops lavender oil
1 drop eucalyptus oil
1 drop rosemary oil
20 ml base oil

Use some before you leave, after your aromatic bath, and take the remainder with you. Whenever you feel discomfort on your travels, find a private space and apply the mixture to your legs, arms and lower back.

Air Travel

Flying tends to put stress on all our senses. Dehydration, anxiety, aches, dry skin, headaches, swollen ankles and a bloated stomach are manifestations of our body trying to adjust to being in a pressurized environment. Aromatherapy can help the adjustment process along, as the key to a stress-free flight is to be as relaxed as possible.

Prepare yourself with an aromatic bath or shower which can prevent the above symptoms from manifesting in the first place, and place you in a very relaxed frame of mind. Try the following pre-flight bath formula:

> 3 drops geranium oil
> 2 drops lavender oil
> 2.5 ml base oil

Once you have had a thorough soaking, massage your body with the following body rub, paying attention to stress points such as the forehead, temples, sinuses, neck, stomach, lower back and ankles:

> 1 drop chamomile oil
> 2 drops geranium oil
> 1 drop lavender oil
> 20 ml base oil

This formula has the added bonus of moisturizing your skin. The pressurized aircabin can leave you feeling parched and dehydrated throughout the journey so drink plenty of fluids before and during the flight, but avoid alcohol and coffee. You can make an excellent refresher spray for your face by filling a small spray bottle with distilled water and/or rosewater and adding a drop of geranium oil.

Attempting to sleep during a long-haul flight can be a task in itself, but inhaling from a tissue or handkerchief scented with a drop of lavender oil can help you to drift away.

Anxiety

Familiarity and security go hand in hand, so you may feel anxious when in unfamiliar surroundings. Aromatherapy can help you cope with such feelings. If you use essential oils regularly, the aromas will provide a sense of comfort wherever you are. Children are particularly vulnerable to feelings of insecurity or homesickness when away from home, even if it is only for a short vacation. You can dispel their fears by using essential oils to provide an ambience of security and comfort. A few drops of essential oil added to bath water or to a vapour ring on a night-light can ensure that there will be no tears before bedtime.

Use this formula for a relaxing aromatic bath for children:

1 drop chamomile oil or
1 drop lavender oil or
1 drop geranium oil
2.5 ml base oil

Adults manifest anxiety as a result of stressful situations and demands which go hand in hand with modern living. Panic attacks, shallow breathing, difficulties in sleeping and short tempers can occur during your holiday. Being away from the demands of the office only to find them replaced by the responsibilities of organizing the annual family trip can be a strain to say the least. Make the most of your time away by enjoying relaxing, aromatic baths during the evenings. Try this formula:

2 drops chamomile oil
2 drops lavender oil
2.5 ml base oil

Burning up to five drops of lavender oil in a vapour ring before bedtime aids a restful sleep.

Arrival

After a long journey, you can rejuvenate yourself with essential oils. To prepare yourself for arrival, clear your head and enliven your senses, place a drop of lavender oil on your fingertips and massage your temples for a minute or two in a clockwise direction.

Before disembarking, make your way to the bathroom and fill a basin with lukewarm water. Add one drop of lavender oil and agitate the water to disperse the essences. Splash your face a few times with the aromatic solution and you will feel pleasantly awake and refreshed.

Follow the floral wash with a breath freshener. Add one drop of peppermint oil to a cupful of water (disposable beakers are provided on all commercial flights) and gargle the contents thoroughly to rinse teeth and gums. This simple routine works wonders every time.

When you return from holiday it can take up to a week to adjust to what was once so familiar. Essential oils can quickly bring you back to 'reality' by stimulating your relaxed senses to a state of awareness. Once back at home or in the office, inhale regularly from a tissue or handkerchief scented with a drop of peppermint or rosemary oil.

Atmosphere

You can use essential oils to create a healthy atmosphere around you – wherever you are. This sound
self-help practice will make you less vulnerable to
airborne bacteria which can be found in unfamiliar
surroundings such as hostel dormitories. Essential
oils are an excellent alternative to commercially
manufactured air-fresheners: not only are they
pleasantly fragranced, they also have antibacterial
and antiviral properties which purify the air.
Furthermore, they do not cause allergic reactions
when inhaled and they do not contain CFCs (chlorofluorocarbons) which deplete the ozone layer.

While travelling, you can purify your surroundings with a convenient essential-oil air-freshener.
You will need five drops of essential oil. Use just one
oil or a blend of five, choosing from the following:

- *geranium*
- *lavender*
- *lemongrass*
- *rosemary*
- *tea tree*

Add the essential oil to a spray bottle containing 100
ml (20 tablepoons) of distilled water and shake vigorously. Spray into the air, towards carpets and cur-
tains (essential oils do not stain but may mark silk
so avoid this material). You may, however, prefer
to use a vapour ring (*see page* 15). Mix five drops of

oil with a little water, then pour into the groove provided.

While camping, sprinkle five to ten drops onto log fires for an agreeable aromatic experience. You can choose essences that encourage a restful sleep or repel night insects, and enjoy experimenting with combinations that are pleasurable to your senses.

Backache

After a long day sailing or hiking with a backpack – or even after awkwardly stepping out of a car – backache can afflict you without warning. A soothing hot compress steeped in essential oils can ease pain in the lower-back area. Add the following formula to a bowl of hot water:

> 1 drop eucalyptus oils
> 1 drop peppermint oil
> 1 drop rosemary oil
> 5 ml base oil

Soak a flannel with the liquid, squeeze it semi-dry then apply it to the lower back. Replace the compress with a freshly soaked flannel as soon as it begins to cool. You may find that two applications a day are necessary for an effective treatment.

Massage eases any back discomfort. Use the following massage oil, and apply with upward and outward movements to stimulate circulation and ensure that the oils are soaked up by the skin:

> 1 drop chamomile oil
> 1 drop rosemary oil
> 10 ml base oil

Essential oils penetrate strained muscle tissue and encourage blood flow which allows regeneration to take place. While treating this area, bend from the knees, keeping your back as straight as possible, and avoid any strenuous movements.

Backpacking
(*see also* CAMPING)

Backpacking through a foreign land is an adventure in itself, a great test of your ability to survive somewhere different with only the basics. It is also a time when you may find yourself staying in some suspect places, many of which have played host to plenty before you. Essential oils, with their antibacterial and antiviral properties, can be your insurance against bringing back unwanted mementoes.

On arrival, sprinkle a few drops of lavender or tea tree oil onto your bedding to ensure restful sleep and keep any bed bugs at bay. Use the following antiviral bath/shower formula during your travels to build up your defences to infection:

> 3 drops eucalyptus oil
> 1 drop lavender oil
> 1 drop tea tree oil
> 2.5 ml base oil

Follow your bath with this delightfully refreshing massage body rub which also has insect-repellent and stimulating properties to help prepare you for the day's events:

> 1 drop eucalyptus oil
> 2 drops lemongrass oil
> 1 drop peppermint oil
> 20 ml base oil

If there is any body rub left, take it with you for use throughout the day.

Bruises

Activity holidays, such as trekking, watersports or skiing, usually invite the odd bruise or two, especially if you are a beginner! There is nothing more unsightly or painful than your souvenir bruise, so attend to it immediately to reduce swelling, discoloration or bedtime soreness.

First, make a cold compress by wrapping ice cubes in a washcloth and apply to affected area. Then mix up the following formula, pour onto the cloth and reapply to bruise:

1 drop chamomile oil
1 drop lavender oil
10 ml base oil

Bees

Bees and wasps have evolved differently but administer the same sting, which is a poison. Bumblebees are mainly found in temperate regions of Asia, Europe and North America, although they can also be found in smaller numbers in Siberia, Greenland and Alaska. There are few bumblebees in the tropics as this is the domain of the honeybee and the wasp. The UK has both types of bee, but bumblebees are predominant.

Generally speaking, bumblebees will sting only if they are provoked or their nests are under attack. Likewise, a wasp stings only in self-defence or to paralyse prey. Only the females of both species are capable of stinging. The female reproductive system in insects opens into a pore near the tip of the abdomen where a needle-like tube is extended and eggs are laid. Bees and wasps have a modification to this structure, which no longer serves a reproductive function. The shaft of the bumblebee, like that of the wasp, is able to penetrate the skin and inject poison, then withdraw from the target. Honeybees, however, have a series of thorns attached to their sting resulting in the whole sting being ripped from the tip of the bees' body once they inject poison and attempt to fly away.

Stings are painful and distressing. The alkaline poison is injected from two sacs just inside the rear end of the bee or wasp. In some cases, this can result in temporary paralysis of the stung area (although smaller creatures react by going into a prolonged coma).

If you are stung by a honeybee sting, you should try to remove the barb. Small tweezers come in handy. Wash the sting and surrounding area with the following antiseptic aromatic solution:

> 1 drop eucalyptus oil
> 2 drops lavender oil
> 1 drop tea tree oil
> 100 ml warm water

After washing, make up the following solution and apply to the skin as often as needed throughout the day:

> 3–5 drops lavender oil
> 1 teaspoon lemon juice

The acidity in this solution counteracts the alkaline sting.

Burns

(*see also* SUNBURN)

Although campfires are inviting, they are one of the main sources of burns on holiday. If you are unsure about how to build a campfire, enlist the help of a park warden or a more experienced fellow camper and be sure to keep an eye on children.

Some burns necessitate immediate medical attention so contact the emergency services as soon as possible. In the meantime, apply ice or cold water to the area for at least 10 minutes to cool the burn and prevent blisters. Then dry the wound. Under no circumstances apply any oil-based product. Follow the cooling process with applications of neat lavender essential oil, using no more than five drops at a time, and wait until it evaporates before reapplying. Apply as often as needed and try to keep the area dry. If the burn causes discomfort at night, apply neat lavender oil to a dry cotton compress and cover the affected area.

Lavender reduces the risk of infection and stimulates the regeneration of the skin to heal with minimal scarring.

Camping

There is nothing like experiencing the great out-doors in a secure, comfortable tent. Essential oils are invaluable here in preventing bugs from spoiling your enjoyment. To repel insects, suspend a vapour ring, to which you have added water, over a portable light, then add the following oils:

> 1 drop eucalyptus oil
> 3 drops lemongrass oil
> 1 drop peppermint oil

Alternatively, mix the oils with 100 ml (20 tea-spoons) of water and spray your pitch, remember-ing to shake the bottle vigorously to disperse the essences throughout the water first. The ideal time to do this is on arrival; the insects will literally clear the area so you can set up your tent without the risk of bugs invading equipment and bedding.

Wipe the inside and outside of your tent with the above formula. Sprinkle three to five drops of lemongrass or lavender oil (or a combination) neat onto your bedding; this prevents unwanted visita-tions from bed bugs and ensures a restful sleep. The above formula has a multitude of other uses. An excellent disinfectant, it can be used in the same dilution for wiping food-storage containers and table tops.

When venturing out for a day's hike, apply the following massage-oil formula to exposed parts of your skin. This will deter bugs, encourage circulation to prevent muscular strains, deodorize the body and clear the head. The sesame base oil acts as a natural sun filter:

1 drop eucalyptus oil
2 drops lemongrass oil
1 drop peppermint oil
20 ml sesame base oil

Start the day with a refreshing bath or shower using this anti-viral bath formula:

2 drops eucalyptus oil
1 drop lavender oil
1 drop tea tree oil
2.5 ml base oil

Chamomile
(see page 20)

Chapped Lips

Extreme weather conditions or a change in body temperature can result in dry, flaky or chapped skin. The lips are often affected first. To keep them smooth and supple, apply the following formula day and night:

> 1 drop chamomile oil
> 1 drop lavender oil
> 10 ml base oil

This amount will last for a few days and can be applied as often as needed. For convenience, decant the mixture into a small phial. You will find that, apart from hydrating your lips, the essences serve as a delightful breath freshener.

The above formula can be doubled and used as an all-over body rub in the case of excessively dry skin. Remember to double the base oil as well as the essential oil dosage (*see Quick Reference Chart, page 123*).

Children

Children love aromas so you will have no trouble finding willing participants for a body rub. While travelling, take care to store essential oils out of their reach.

The aromatherapy formulas in this book are meant for adults, unless otherwise specified. Children can still benefit from aromatherapy, however, but smaller dosages are more compatible with their physiological and psychological development. Lavender, chamomile and geranium oils are all suitable for use on babies and children under the age of 12. For topical application, the dosage should be one drop of essential oil to every 15 ml of base oil; for use in the bath, one drop of essential oil should be mixed with 5 ml of base oil; for a floral spray wash, use one drop of essential oil in 200 ml of distilled water and shake vigorously before use; and in vapour rings, use a maximum of two drops of essence (eucalyptus oil can be used for children suffering from colds or fevers). For more information on using essential oils on children, *see ANXIETY*.

Colds

There is no cure as yet for the common cold, but many symptoms can be alleviated with the help of aromatherapy. Prepare an aromatic bath with the following formula, and inhale the vapours deeply while relaxing:

> 3 drops eucalyptus oil
> 2 drops geranium oil
> 2.5 ml base oil

Make up the following formula and use it to massage around your sinuses, paying attention to your nose, cheekbones and forehead. Then use it to massage your neck and chest:

> 1 drop eucalyptus oil
> 1 drop rosemary oil
> 10 ml base oil

Blocked sinuses can be dealt with by placing a drop or two of eucalyptus oil on a tissue or handkerchief and inhaling whenever you feel it necessary.

Carry out the above treatments daily, and continue for three days after the symptoms have subsided. This simple yet effective routine will provide much relief by helping you to breathe more easily and regulating your body temperature; and it will also prevent the spread of infection.

Constipation

A very uncomfortable and embarrassing ailment, especially when travelling, constipation should be addressed as soon as possible. Constipation can occur as a result of anxiety – especially during air travel – or can be caused by your body adjusting to unfamiliar foods. Ideally, find a private space and massage your abdomen in a clockwise direction with the following formula:

> 1 drop rosemary oil
> 1 drop peppermint oil
> 10 ml base oil

If the constipation is a prolonged condition, there could be an underlying cause. Check your dietary habits: no matter where you are in the world, you should be eating plenty of wholegrains and green, leafy vegetables, and maintaining a high fluid intake. If symptoms persist and develop into chronic pain, consult the local doctor.

Cramp

Cramp can be very painful. It can occur after intense physical activity such as hiking, watersports or skiing, and also as a result of dehydration. After suffering from a bout of cramp, replenish fluids immediately by drinking at least a litre of water to which you have added a teaspoon of salt. Continue drinking throughout the day, as you will probably find yourself unusually thirsty.

A hot compress relaxes the tense muscle and encourages blood flow. To make one, dip a flannel in medium-hot water then squeeze out the excess liquid before applying to the affected muscle.

Massaging the muscle with firm pressure can help by encouraging circulation. Use the following formula:

1 drop eucalyptus oil
1 drop geranium oil
10 ml base oil

Cuts

In the event of a cut, the priority is to lessen the risk of infection, particularly in areas of the world where the climate is tropical or humid. All essential oils have powerful antibacterial and antiseptic properties yet are safe to use on the skin when diluted in the correct amount of base oil. They are less 'stinging' than commercial disinfectants and encourage the healing process. Bathe the area with warm water (100 ml) to which you have added:

> 2 drops lavender oil
> 1 drop tea tree oil
> 2.5 ml base oil

Dry the area then apply three to five drops of neat lavender oil to the wound and cover with a dry compress – a small piece of gauze or a handkerchief will do. If you do this daily, you will find that the cut heals quickly. You can aid healing by airing the cut once you notice scar tissue mending.

Driving

Aromatherapy is an essential aid to driving. A bold statement to make, perhaps, but not unreasonable when one considers the increased and sustained level of clarity and concentration that can be induced while driving by using rosemary essential oil. Whether it is a long journey across country or a short trip across town, rosemary has a remarkable effect on the nervous system. A mental and physical stimulant, it literally clears your head and is great for improving memory.

A pomander (cloth or terracotta) and a few drops of rosemary oil are all you need to create a useful car accessory. Pomanders can be bought in health-food shops or, if you feel creative, you can make your own from a natural sponge and cloth. The cost is minimal and the effect is well worth it. Add five drops of rosemary oil to your pomander and replenish every other week. The pomander is also an excellent car freshener and a great alternative to the commercial varieties which are impregnated with artificial fragrances. Stepping into a herbal car is quite refreshing and the essence has an added bonus of counteracting smoke and exhaust fumes which can infiltrate your vehicle (*see also* POLLUTION).

Dysentery

Dysentery is a highly infectious, extremely uncomfortable condition, causing diarrhoea with blood and mucus and abdominal pain. The bacteria are carried by contaminated water, in food not properly washed or cooked and by flies in tropical destinations. Preventive measures are of paramount importance.

Garlic capsules (*see* GARLIC) are indispensable here as they purify the blood and encourage your internal organs to fight unfriendly bacteria. Two capsules per day are sufficient to build resistance, but they are most effective when taken over a long period of time. A month before your journey, increase your intake to three capsules per day, and continue with this dosage for a further two weeks once you return home.

There is not much you can do to ensure food is properly cooked (except for cooking it yourself!), but you should drink plenty of bottled or cooled, boiled water. Even when bathing or washing, use cooled, boiled water. The following disinfectant wash formula comes in extremely handy:

1 drop eucalyptus oil
2 drops lavender oil
1 drop tea tree
100 ml distilled water

Shake the bottle vigorously. Each time you wash, add 50 ml of the solution to the water. For bathing, add the essential oils to 5 ml of base oil before mixing with bath water. The same dosage can be diluted in 20 ml of base oil as a body rub. Regularly used, the above formulas act as powerful antiviral aids, yet are also refreshing and uplifting in a hot climate.

If the worst happens and you become infected with dysentery, consult a doctor, as saline injections may need to be prescribed. Given the infectious nature of the bacteria, you will have to be isolated. Cheer yourself up by spraying the room with 3 drops of lavender or rosemary essential oil diluted in 100 ml of distilled water, or use a vapour ring to diffuse the essences. Continue your dosage of garlic capsules. Muscle pain may occur as your body attempts to rebalance itself, so massage yourself daily with the body rub formula. For accompanying headaches, apply a drop of neat lavender oil to the temples, massaging in a clockwise direction, and along the base of your skull (the occipital ridge).

Eucalyptus
(see page 21)

Eye Care

Tired eyes are a physical manifestation of long-haul travel. Some companies supply eye-care packs for travellers (*see Retailers and Suppliers, page* 152). There are also a number of do-it-yourself aromatherapy methods.

If you have included chamomile tea bags in your travel kit, place one over each eye after dipping them in lukewarm water and squeezing out the excess liquid. Alternatively, a cool compress can soothe swollen, red, puffy eyes. Dip a piece of gauze or a cotton wool pad in ice-cold water and place over the eye area for a minute or two. You may like to splash your face first with 1 drop of lavender oil diluted in 2 litres of water. Leave the compress in position for five minutes and relax.

Applying a drop of vitamin E oil or almond oil to the eye area can also benefit tired eyes and soften the skin around them. Dotting the oil around the brow area and the rim of the eye socket is sufficient to lubricate the whole eye area. Absorb excess oil with a tissue, taking care not to drag the delicate skin.

Fainting

Losing consciousness due to trauma, panic or heat exhaustion requires immediate action. First, loosen tight clothing but do not sit the person up. Take the following steps to get him or her into the recovery position:

1) Turn the person onto his or her right side.
2) Bend up the left leg and lay it across the right leg, which should be straight.
3) Place the left arm at a right angle to the body while the right arm stays down by the side.

Check that the respiratory tract is clear (removing false teeth if necessary). Raise the person's legs higher than the head with anything that can act as a bolster or cushion; this action ensures that the blood continues to flow towards the brain and heart, and breathing resumes as normal. Practise this routine with a willing participant before setting off on your travels as you never know when you may be required to use it.

A powerful nerve stimulant such as peppermint or rosemary oil can be used to activate the fainted person's senses. Hold the bottle directly under the nose or add a drop or two of the essence to a tissue or handkerchief and encourage deep inhalation of the vapours.

If fainting is due to heat exhaustion, replenish fluids as quickly as possible by drinking a litre of salted (1 teaspoon) water (*see also* SUNSTROKE).

Feet

Our feet and legs provide locomotion, enabling us to hop from one flight to another and perform more demanding tasks such as hiking. Taking care of them is a must. The feet house endings of the sciatic nerve – the largest nerve in the body – which runs from the sacrum in our lower back down through our legs. Massaging the feet stimulates these nerve endings – also known as acupressure points – and is pleasurable and relaxing.

Many travellers suffer from swollen ankles and feet due to excess fluid accumulating in the tissues of this area. This can be caused by sitting for long periods, especially in the pressurized atmosphere of an aeroplane. Prepare for such a situation by mixing the following foot-rub formula in advance:

> 1 drop eucalyptus oil
> 1 drop lavender oil
> 10 ml base oil

Spread the oil over and under the feet. Massage firmly with kneading movements towards the legs, concentrating on your toes and ankles for a soothing experience. Remove excess oil with a tissue.

This formula can also be used in preparation for a hike, as the essences stimulate circulation and deodorize. Be sure to wear thick, padded socks and appropriate boots for added comfort. After a hike, foot soaks are wonderfully relaxing. Fill a bowl with hot, but not boiling, water and add a drop or two of geranium, lavender or peppermint oil. Follow your soak with a foot rub by an aromatic campfire for a great ending to the day.

Fever

Fevers developed while travelling are usually a result of a viral or bacterial infection, and tend to be accompanied by a cold or bout of flu. These infections are commonly picked up in tropical climates where they are transmitted by insect bites or in contaminated water supplies.

A feverish body experiences a rise in normal body temperature (37° Celsius/98° Fahrenheit) and fluctuates between extremes of hot and cold with intense sweating and sometimes delirium. The patient must be kept in bed, preferably wrapped in a cotton sheet which allows the body to breathe. Regularly applying a cool compress will help reduce body temperature. To make an aromatic fever compress, first make up the following aromatic formula:

> 1 drop eucalyptus oil
> 1 drop lemongrass oil
> 5 ml base oil

Pour the solution into a bowl (1 litre) of cool water. Dip a flannel or small towel into the water, wring semi-dry and apply to the forehead, neck, chest and, especially, the face.

You can also help to reduce body temperature by adding the following solution to a tepid bath:

1 drop chamomile oil
1 drop eucalyptus oil
2 drops lemongrass oil
2.5 ml base oil

If you are looking after someone with a fever, it is a wise precaution to use the above formula yourself to protect your body from the virus.

While the patient is recovering, burning the following solution in a vapour ring will help purify the air:

4 drops lavender oil
1 drop tea tree
small amount of water

Alternatively, pour the above formula into a 50-ml spray bottle and periodically mist the room. Encourage the patient to drink plenty of water and chamomile tea to replenish lost fluids and flush out toxins.

Fish Bites

Some marine creatures, such as jellyfish and stingrays, produce poisons and venoms. These lethal substances are used for killing or paralysing prey, and some also act as digestive fluids. They are produced by glands found near spines, tentacles, fangs and other piercing apparatus.

Encounters with poisonous fish are most likely to occur when swimming in shallow waters or rivers, where some creatures are easily camouflaged by embedding themselves within the sand and river beds. Jellyfish have the added advantage of being able to creep up on their intended victim by being difficult to detect with their translucent blue, pink or violet bodies.

Like all jellyfish, the Portuguese man-of-war can be found in the warm seas throughout the world. It is most common in the tropical and sub-tropical areas of the Indian and Pacific Oceans and the north Atlantic Ocean. The translucent, gas-filled, circular body can have tentacles beneath of up to 50 metres (165 feet) in length, each capable of stinging with a dose of poison. Apart from the sting being very painful, the poison results in shock and breathing difficulties, progressing to fever and heart palpitations.

Stingrays are flat-bodied fish which can also be found in the warm climates, mainly congregating in shallow coastal areas and rivers. They have a tendency to bury themselves partially, so they can be very difficult to spot. Their long, sharp spines cause very painful wounds, and the poison administered can result in acute abdominal reactions.

When using essential oils to counteract a fish bite, it is important to bear in mind that such treatment takes second priority to seeking urgent medical attention. Essential oils are, however, invaluable in providing immediate first aid. If you are about to set off on a holiday which will involve swimming in rivers or the sea, prepare a small (100 ml) bottle of a powerful antiviral, antiseptic, disinfectant wash using the following formula:

2 drops lavender oil
1 drop peppermint oil
1 drop tea tree oil
2.5 ml base oil

Add the mixture to 100 ml of water, and shake the bottle before each use. Dab the bite with a cotton wool pad that has been soaked in the solution. Apply five drops of neat lavender oil to the bite and reapply the solution, if necessary, as soon as the previous dose has been absorbed by the skin. Keep up this procedure until you arrive at the hospital.

Floral Waters

Floral waters are essential oils suspended in distilled water, mineral water, rosewater or combinations of the three. They can be used as disinfectants, tonics, body coolers, facial rinses and mouthwashes. The solutions have to be shaken vigorously to disperse the oils throughout the water, and should be used immediately afterwards. This is because alcohol – a standard diffusing agent – is not added to the solution. Even in minute quantities, alcohol can be irritating to some skin types or conditions, and it is not a practical addition to a travelling kit.

Formulas vary from one drop of essential oil suspended in 200 ml of water for a toner to five drops per 100 ml in the case of a powerful disinfectant. Many types of floral water are described in this book, and they are best used via a spray bottle for convenience while travelling. (*See also Quick Reference Chart, page* 123).

Food Poisoning
(*see* DYSENTERY *and* UPSET STOMACH)

Frostbite

Frostbite occurs when you have been exposed to extreme cold, in conditions such as those found at altitudes above 2500 metres (8000 feet). Apart from the inability to feel sensation in your body, you may experience periodical itchiness as your metabolism and circulation attempt to adjust to the exterior influence of the low temperature. This may result in chilblains (particularly on the hands and feet) and fluctuations in body temperature. Chilblains manifest as swelling of the joints, discoloration of the skin and extremely uncomfortable itching sensations. Massage the affected area with this warming blend:

> 1 drop *eucalyptus oil*
> 2 drops *geranium oil*
> 1 drop *rosemary oil*
> 20 ml *base oil*

Ensure you warm your body as soon as possible by putting on several layers of clothing.

Garlic

Garlic can benefit your health in many ways. Odourless capsules are available which contain minute quantities of garlic essential oil suspended in a vegetable oil base and encapsulated in gelatine. Packed with vitamins A, B and C, the capsules also have a high content of the minerals calcium, phosphorous, iron, sodium and potassium.

Garlic capsules are indispensable in preventing all sorts of problems. For urinary disorders, garlic is as excellent diuretic, and it is effective against worms, infections, coughs and as an expectorant. The capsules dissolve in the stomach, enter the bloodstream and circulate the entire body, eradicating harmful bacteria and healing skin disorders. Taken regularly, garlic purifies and strengthens the blood, tones the heart and liver and aids digestive processes.

Taking two capsules a day for at least a month prior to travelling should provide adequate protection against transmittable infections for most climates. When travelling to a climate where there may be contaminated water supplies, however, increase the dosage to three capsules. (*See* DYSENTERY.)

You can buy garlic capsules in health-food shops or pharmacies and, apart from their remarkable health-giving benefits, they are extremely cost-effective.

Geranium
(see page 22)

Grazes
(see CUTS)

Hair Care

The condition of your hair can suffer when travelling. Each hair is covered in a protein called keratin which ensures a healthy gloss, body and elasticity. Exposing hair to sun, sea or chlorine in swimming pools weakens the keratin bonding process and can result in dryness, split ends and dullness. Avoid using harsh, detergent-based products. Choose vegetable-based alternatives which are gentle on the hair and scalp. There are a few companies that do not use petrochemicals in their formulas (*see Retailers and Suppliers*).

Essential oils enhance the condition of any hair type due to their exceptional penetrative abilities. Acting as building blocks to the hair, they tone the scalp and encourage healthy hair growth. Adding essential oils to your preferred vegetable-based hair products greatly enhances their conditioning capabilities, thereby addressing imbalances in the condition of the hair and scalp. Your hair will smell great too. Once you have created your custom-blended hair cleansers and conditioners you can decant them into travel containers. Try the following formula for dry hair or scalp:

5 drops rosemary oil
2 drops chamomile oil
2 drops lavender oil
100 ml shampoo/conditioner base

This formula is for oily hair or scalp:

> 3 drops rosemary oil
> 5 drops geranium oil
> 1 drop eucalyptus oil
> 100 ml shampoo/conditioner base

While out and about or swimming, protect your hair with the following anti-sun/chlorine formula:

> 2 drops rosemary oil
> 1 drop chamomile oil
> 1 drop lavender oil
> 1 drop geranium oil
> 20 ml base oil

The above formula can also be used in a larger dosage on dry hair as a pre-conditioning treatment. Use a teaspoon at a time for coating hair ends and scalp. This is an ideal time to massage your scalp with the pads of your fingers to stimulate blood flow and loosen a tight scalp. Be sure to move the scalp and not the skin; applying a slight pressure to your scalp is the key. You will find 10 minutes of circular movements to your scalp a relaxing and pleasant addition to your shampooing routine. The amount of hair oil will vary with regards to hair type and condition but as a general guide:

1–2 teaspoons for short to medium hair
2–3 teaspoons for medium to long hair
3–4 teaspoons long/extremely dry or damaged hair

Apply shampoo directly to the hair to ensure removal of the hair protector. Rinse thoroughly, then lather once more. Apply your aromatic conditioner to hair and scalp, particularly to your hair ends, and leave for 10 minutes to ensure a deep conditioning treatment.

Finish your hair-care routine by rinsing with the following floral wash which seals cuticles and enhances colour:

1 drop rosemary oil (for dark hair) or
1 drop chamomile oil (for fair or dry hair)

Fill a bowl or jug (of 1 litre capacity) with warm water and add the relevant essential oil. Stir the solution to disperse the essence through the water then pour over your hair and scalp.

By the end of your trip, your hair will be in tip-top condition.

Hayfever

An allergic reaction to pollen, hayfever can afflict anyone, often without warning. The runny nose, incessant sneezing and general discomfort can mar any trip abroad. Essential oils, however, can come to the rescue, balancing nature with nature.

Place a drop of chamomile oil and a drop of lemongrass oil on a tissue or handkerchief and sniff to alleviate symptoms. Massage the chest, sinuses and neck with the following formula:

> 1 drop chamomile oil
> 1 drop lemongrass oil
> 1 drop tea tree oil
> 15 ml base oil

A teaspoon of the above can also be added to baths until the condition ceases.

Headaches

Holiday headaches can knock you off balance and prevent you from enjoying yourself to the full. Varying in duration and pressure, they can be caused by sunstroke, stress or eating unfamiliar foods. They can also be related to the hormonal shift experienced during premenstrual tension or to a build up of toxins within the body. Many pharmaceutical manufacturers look to synthetically derived 'quick fixes', but essential oils are effective in soothing pain naturally.

A drop or two of neat lavender oil applied directly to the temples and massaged with a slight pressure in a clockwise direction brings relief across the forehead and bridge of the brow. Toxins tend to accumulate at a gap between the base of the skull and neck (called the occipital ridge) so massaging here can provide rapid relief by dislodging the toxins, which create the tension and pressure felt across the whole head. Drink plenty of water to help flush the toxins through your body once they have been dislodged. Massage with the formula below, paying attention to this area, and across the forehead, cheeks, neck and chest with the pads of your fingertips:

1 drop lavender oil
1 drop peppermint oil
10 ml base oil

An aromatic bath certainly helps, so prepare the following formula:

> 3 drops lavender oil
> 2 drops rosemary oil
> 2.5 ml base oil

Remember to inhale the vapours deeply and, if it is bedtime, apply the headache formula before you retire to encourage a restful sleep.

Heat Exhaustion
(*see* SUNSTROKE)

Indigestion

During flights you may experience flatulence or indigestion. Although this is embarrassing, rest assured that you are definitely not alone. Your stomach may feel bloated due to the expansion of gases brought about by being in a pressurized cabin. Eating unfamiliar foods can result in indigestion, and peppermint is a useful ally in relieving discomfort. In acute cases of flatulence or indigestion, the following blend should be applied to the abdomen and lower back:

1 drop peppermint oil
1 drop rosemary oil
10 ml base oil

Massage with a slow, clockwise motion using the flat of your hands to ensure penetration of the essences and dispersion of accumulated gases.

Following the treatment, drink plenty of hot water and eat small amounts of easily digested foods such as soups and live yoghurt until your system regains balance.

Insect Bites
(see also Appendix 1 and MOSQUITO BITES)

No other form of life can match the diversity of insects. The majority of mites inhabit soil or surface vegetation, feeding on plant and animal remains or faeces. They prefer to dwell where there is an abundance of moisture, such as in forests, meadows and lakeside areas. Some of these little creatures enter into co-habitation arrangements with animals, although the arrangement is not mutual where we are concerned!

Like all social living creatures, the main business of the mite is to gain food from its hosts in the form of sebaceous secretions, although being transported from one place to another by a large animal has its attractions. In contrast to lice and fleas, bed bugs are fairly recent cosmopolitan travellers. They are now widespread due to being transported all over the world by people and their belongings.

There is more to an overfriendly insect than its bite. Scratching a bite can cause infection, and there is also the threat of the spread of disease. The spread of the bubonic plague or 'Black Death' through Europe, which wiped out a quarter of the population, was attributed not only to rats, but also to the fleas that lived on them and continued to spread the disease once their host had died.

Most of us are unaware of having been bitten, since it is painless at the time and more likely to occur during sleep. Once bitten, there are two distinct skin reactions:

1) The immediate reaction, which occurs in a few minutes,
   subsiding within an hour.
2) The delayed reaction, which manifests as swelling, irritation
   and reddening of the affected area, usually lasting for a few
   days.

The good news is that an allergic reaction to the bite
is a sign of your body doing its best to manufacture
an antibody to the intruding germs and toxins.

While travelling in the tropics, insect-repellent is
essential. Commercial repellents claim to be effective, but I and many other travellers have found them
of little use. Apart from this, the synthetic ingredi-
ents and chlorofluorocarbon gases (CFCs) in most
commercial brands can harm the environment.
When I was travelling in the West Indies, I found
myself attracting bugs left, right and centre.
Travellers to a climate unlike their own will not have
acquired the immunity which comes with genera-
tions of living in tropical and sub-tropical climates.
Travellers or newcomers to the land are therefore
more likely to suffer incessant biting. I therefore
spent time formulating the ideal environmentally
friendly insect-repellent, adopting a routine which
quite successfully kept them at bay.

Make a floral water of the following essences
which you will find effective in repelling insects in
your vicinity. You will find the aromas uplifting and
refreshing in a tropical or sub-tropical climate:

1 drop eucalyptus oil
3 drops lemongrass oil
1 drop peppermint oil
1 drop tea tree oil
100 ml (spray bottle) distilled water

The formula should be shaken vigorously before spraying. The chemical components of the essential oils, notably citrol and eucalyptol, are offensive to bed bugs, fleas, mites, sandflies and mosquitoes. The formula can be sprayed on to bedding, carpets and clothing (except silk) as well as into the air.

The above essential oils – minus tea tree – can also be applied topically in the form of a body rub after a bath or shower:

1 drop eucalyptus oil
2 drops lemongrass oil
1 drop peppermint oil
20 ml base oil

The formula can be applied liberally, paying attention to the ankles, a favourite target for insects.

To ensure a peaceful and insect-free night's sleep, prepare your sleeping area in advance by dispensing the following formula in a vapour ring or water bowl:

2 drops lavender oil
3 drops lemongrass oil

The following disinfectant is useful for alleviating symptoms from bites and stings from bees, wasps, gnats, sandflies, waterticks and fleas (for mosquito bites, see separate entry).

1 drop eucalyptus oil
2 drops lavender oil
1 drop tea tree oil
100 ml water

Add the oils to the water and shake vigorously to disperse them. Swab the affected area then apply three to five drops of neat lavender oil every half hour for four hours until swelling subsides. If this does not happen, the spread of infection may not have been caught in time and a visit to the doctor is necessary.

Insomnia

Children, in particular, are prone to insomnia when away from home. In recent years, however, the business traveller has been increasingly susceptible to this manifestation of stress. Corporate competitiveness has intensified, and the business traveller leads a stressful life, jumping on and off planes, preparing documents for various meetings and being expected to make a good enough impression to win the confidence of a client or clinch a deal.

To work efficiently, you need to be in good form, both mentally and physically. You can achieve this by combating stress with a relaxing regime of aromatherapy. Once you arrive at your destination or prior to bedtime, prepare an aromatic bath by adding the following essences to a tub of medium-hot water:

1 drop chamomile oil

3 drops lavender oil

2.5 ml base oil

(For children, use only one drop of either essential oil.) This bath is for relaxing, not cleansing, so take a shower before soaking in the bath for at least 20 minutes. Both these essential oils have a sedative effect, eradicating symptoms of stress and preparing the body for a sound sleep. Inhale the vapours deeply while relaxing and capitalize on this time by focusing on anything except business – perhaps the sound of your breathing or soothing music. In fact, try to think of nothing except your relaxing bath.

Apply a drop of neat lavender oil to a corner of your pillow so that you inhale the relaxing vapour as you sleep.

Jet-lag

A modern phenomenon which accompanies air travel, jet-lag is not only uncomfortable and disorientating but can also take up valuable time which could be better spent at your holiday destination or on business. Whether you travel from north to south or east to west, jet-lag can occur as your sensory system adjusts to high-speed travelling and a new time zone and environment. Such influences can disturb up to 50 physiological and psychological body rhythms. Aware of such disruption, many airlines now monitor their staff's biorhythms before drawing up rotas.

Essential oils can alleviate symptoms of jet-lag such as fatigue, nervousness and irritability. Before embarking on your journey, prepare a pre-flight aromatic bath with the following formula:

1 drop geranium oil
2 drops lavender oil
1 drop lemongrass oil
2.5 ml base oil

Geranium is an excellent nerve tonic, and helps redress any imbalances in the central nervous system where our sensory perceptions are registered.

If you arrive at your destination ready for bed but find that the local time is not near your usual bedtime, try to stay awake for a few hours, retiring for bed at the time you would if at home. You may find that adding this aromatic combination to bath water aids a restful sleep:

1 drop chamomile oil
1 drop geranium oil
1 drop lavender oil
2.5 ml base oil

If you use this formula in your evening bath for the next three days, you will soon adjust to your new environment. If, however, you have a meeting to attend as soon as you arrive, bathe with the following formula which has an uplifting effect on the senses and results in a wide-awake state:

2 drops eucalyptus oil
1 drop geranium oil
3 drops rosemary oil
2.5 ml base oil

Bathing in the morning with these essences makes for a refreshing start to the day, and you may wish to continue using this formula throughout the trip. The same formula can be used on sponges when showering, but be sure to use the formula as your last rinse as it will not cleanse the body.

Follow each bath with this aromatic body rub, designed to soothe the nerves and relax the mind and body:

2 drops geranium oil
2 drops lavender oil
20 ml base oil

Lavender
(see page 23)

Lemongrass
(see page 25)

Men's Skin

Travelling can play havoc with men's skin. Adventure holidays expose the skin to the elements, and business travel also takes its toll. Added to which is the daily shaving routine, which removes not only the hair but also a layer of the epidermis, leaving the skin tender and prone to inflammation, razor bumps or keloids.

Prior to shaving, prime the skin with the following formula which softens the stubble and protects against the sensitivity experienced after shaving:

> 1 drop chamomile oil
> 5 ml base oil

Smooth the mixture over the area to be shaved, including the neck, then lather with a vegetable-based cream or soap. After your shave, add one drop of eucalyptus oil to a bowl of warm water, then splash the face to tone the skin. Eucalyptus has antiseptic properties and is an excellent deodorizer. Finish by applying some more of the pre-shave formula to maintain suppleness, especially when outdoors (see HIKING).

Mouthwash

Fragrant breath not only feels refreshing but also helps you create a good impression – essential for business travellers. Bad breath may indicate a sluggish digestive system, so check your dietary habits and include more water, fruit and vegetables in your diet. The following mouthwash is essential for travellers as it freshens the breath after eating spicy foods and enlivens anyone suffering from jet-lag. It is very cost-effective and purifying, with antibacterial and antiviral properties that are excellent for cleansing the teeth, gums and tonsils. The formula should be shaken vigorously before each use. You will find 20 ml enough for one wash.

1 drop peppermint oil or
1 drop rosemary oil
200 ml distilled water

Mosquito Bites
(see also Appendix 1 and INSECT BITES)

Hardy mosquitoes have adapted to vaccines and repellents, mutating to such a degree that some of the synthetic products on the market have been rendered ineffective. Though they have a short life-cycle in the tropics (10 days), mosquitoes can live for several months if transported to a cooler region where they multiply – rapidly.

Mosquitoes feast upon blood, travelling from person to person, animal to animal; that is how malaria and yellow fever spread. During the 1990s, malaria has been on the increase in tropical and subtropical climates.

The females require blood to feed and develop their eggs which they lay on the surface of ponds, lakes and even puddles. Attracted to humans and other animals by moisture, perspiration, body heat and movement, mosquitoes rarely deviate from a preferred host, and travellers are most certainly a favourite by bringing an unfamiliar, distinctive blood taste into a region.

Fortunately, essential oils such as lemongrass contain a substance called citrol which is offensive to mosquitoes. When travelling to areas where they are prevalent, arm yourself with the following insect-repellent spray formula:

1 drop eucalyptus oil
3 drops lemongrass oil
1 drop peppermint oil
1 drop tea tree oil
100 ml distilled water

Shake the formula before spraying around your immediate vicinity including bedding, clothing and the air. (For information on further methods of repelling mosquitoes, *see* INSECT-REPELLENTS.)

Garlic capsules (*see page 69*) are also useful for repelling mosquitoes as they contain chemicals offensive to the insects. If you succumb to a bite, wash the affected area with the following antiseptic formula and apply a maximum of five drops of neat lavender oil to the bite. Continue with this treatment until swelling subsides and avoid scratching as much as possible:

1 drop eucalyptus oil
2 drops lemongrass oil
1 drop tea tree oil
100 ml distilled water

Dilute the same formula in 20 ml of base oil and use as a body rub to deter insects. Pay attention to the ankles, arms and face (avoiding the eye area) and reapply during the day.

Muscular Pain

Muscular pain can be unbearable. Interestingly, it can be caused by two opposite extremes: overactivity and underactivity. A highly active person may experience a build-up of lactic acid in the body which leads to pain, and someone who languishes on the beach, barely lifting a finger for two weeks can find that muscle fatigue sets in, also causing pain.

While away on vacation or on business, moderate exercise will ensure your body functions at an optimum level of equilibrium. Time spent practising yoga on the beach or working out in a gym will be a good investment as your body will reap untold benefits in the long term. Your body will thank you for the energy boost and lithe physique.

If you are a highly active person, here is a massage formula which eases pain, increases circulation and disperses lactic acid:

1 drop *eucalyptus oil*
1 drop *lavender oil*
2 drops *rosemary oil*
20 ml *base oil*

Massage towards the heart using long, deep strokes. Maintain contact with the affected muscle until the oil is absorbed by the skin.

Nettle Rash

Nettle rash and other plant stings are extremely uncomfortable and need to be addressed without delay. When wandering out into the wilderness, even the thickest of socks will not necessarily provide adequate protection. Essential oils are useful in emergencies. Wash the area immediately in cold water and apply neat lavender oil (or eucalyptus diluted in 5 ml of base oil) to the stung area. Once back at the base, wash with the antiseptic wash on page 54 and apply the following blend to the sting and surrounding areas:

> 1 drop chamomile oil
> 1 drop tea tree oil
> 10 ml base oil

Reapply as necessary until the reaction subsides.

Nosebleeds

Although nosebleeds can happen to anyone for no apparent reason, children are particularly prone to them. This can be unsettling for both child and parent, especially on holiday. Children tend to panic at the sight of blood, so quick action is needed to address the bleeding and reassure the child.

First, find a convenient place for the child to lie down (if this is not possible, hold the child's head back as far as possible). Pinch just above the bridge of the nose while holding a tissue to the nostrils to which you have added two drops of lavender oil. Encourage the child to inhale the vapours.

Peppermint
(see page 26)

Pollution

Approaching living and travelling with a caring conscience, experiencing other places by adopting a 'leave only footprints, take only memories' attitude, contributes to creating a new appreciation of travel and other cultures.

Swimming in the sea and in rivers is appealing to many holiday-makers, but these days you are more likely to catch an infection than a fish. This is due to the widespread pollution of the world's waters, which have been used as dumping grounds for sewage, radiation, toxic metals and other contaminated substances. Check with the National Forestry Commission, National Trust (or equivalent in the countries you visit) who can recommend areas where there are rivers and streams fit to bathe in. You will find a list of centres in the phone book or you can inquire at tourist offices.

Avoid swimming in lakes or coastal areas where watersports such as jet-skiing or speedboating are popular, as the expelled fuel could affect you adversely. When participating in such sports, wear adequate protective clothing to prevent infection. Suitable attire is available in sports and adventure shops and is a worthwhile investment for your health. If you own or hire a speedboat, choose a 'green' fuel, such as lead-free petrol, if possible (*see also* DRIVING).

Remember to protect your hair with the formula on page 72. After such sports, shower immediately, adding one of these essential oils directly to your sponge or loofah during your final rinse:

3–5 drops eucalyptus oil or
3–5 drops lavender oil

You will be pleased to know that, by using essential oils, you will not be polluting the environment in any way. They are a product of nature and therefore biodegradable. By using essential oils you – as the consumer – will encourage the industry to cultivate more herbs, plants and flowers to meet your demand.

Premenstrual Tension

In recent years, premenstrual tension (also known as premenstrual syndrome) has been recognized by the medical profession as a 'real' manifestation of the hormone imbalance experienced by women during this time. The ratio of the hormones secreted varies from woman to woman. Symptoms include uncontrollable weeping, headaches, uterine cramp, loss of concentration, bloated abdomen, irritability and depression. Cases of suicide have even been recorded where women have been particularly affected by PMT.

Even the most hardened female traveller will feel less than her best if any of these symptoms occur during her holiday or business trip. Fortunately, help is at hand in the form of essential oils. These remarkable essences contain chemicals that stimulate the endocrine system and rectify the imbalance of hormonal secretions. Women and those close to them (mainly their partners) need not suffer every month, for by including essential oils in your health-maintenance routine, your monthly 'curse' can be transformed into a monthly aromatic pampering session which provides relief physically, emotionally and mentally.

Generally speaking, premenstrual tension can last from as much as two weeks to as little as three days before menstruation. It can cease once bleeding occurs or continue for three days afterwards. The best time to start preparing for the inevitable is around ovulation. There are certain signs that let you know when this is happening, such as a rise in body temperature or the appearance of any of the symptoms mentioned above.

Nothing is more relaxing and calming to your nerves than a daily aromatic bath during your premenstrual phase. The following formula eases pain and restores balance to the nervous system:

> 3 drops geranium oil
> 1 drop lavender oil
> 2 drops rosemary
> 2.5 ml base oil

Avoid bathing in hot water but soak in a medium-temperature bath. Follow this with a soothing massage, paying attention to the abdomen, lower back and chest areas. Use the following massage oil formula:

> 2 drops geranium oil
> 2 drops rosemary oil
> 20 ml base oil

Geranium is a powerful nerve tonic which is simultaneously sedating and uplifting. It is used by doctors in Italy to treat anxiety-related conditions. Women prone to weeping or to anxiety attacks will benefit from placing a drop of geranium oil on a tissue or handkerchief and inhaling from it during the course of the day.

Prickly Heat

The term prickly heat refers to heat bumps that spread as a rash, affecting any part of the body and itching uncontrollably. They are caused by the body overheating, resulting in blocked sweat glands. Those particularly affected are travellers unaccustomed to hot climates, mainly children.

The priority here is to reduce the body temperature immediately. This should not, however, be done drastically with cold water, as this could bring about a shock to the nervous system. Apply lukewarm compresses to the body, particularly the face, underarms and top of the head where heat is expired and perspiration is most active. Make up a floral wash in a spray bottle with the following formula:

1 drop *lavender oil*
1 drop *peppermint oil*
5 ml *base oil*
500 ml *distilled water*

Shake the bottle and spray the body with this cooling, aromatic wash. Peppermint evaporates quickly inducing a cooling sensation on the body, while the lavender calms inflamed areas.

Lukewarm baths tend to help reduce temperature slowly and you can prepare a cooling bath with the following blend of essential oils:

2 drops eucalyptus oil
1 drop lavender oil
2.5 ml base oil

For a child, a drop of lavender oil in a lukewarm bath is equally effective at reducing body heat.

Wear loose-fitting cotton clothing so the skin breathes easily and drink plenty of water (adding 1 teaspoon of salt per litre) to prevent dehydration and replenish fluids. (*See also* CHILDREN.)

Rosemary
(see page 27)

Sea Creatures
(see also Appendix 1 and FISH BITES)

Swimming in the sea is a delightful experience and a must for all of us who plan a vacation near a beach. Delight can turn to misery, however, if you find yourself the unlucky recipient of a bite or sting from a sea creature such as a snake, anemone or urchin. Fish bites, though not as unsettling, can cause swelling and illness. In both cases, emergency treatment is a priority. Send for help, and alert the emergency services.

Sea anemones are beautiful marine creatures which curiously resemble flowers. Rather than exude a bouquet, however, they secrete an adhesive which allows them to attach themselves to hard surfaces such as rocks, timber and sea shells. There are up to 1000 different species of sea anemone, varying in size from a few millilitres to 1.5 metres in diameter. Usually yellow, blue or green, anemones can be found from the tidal zone to depths of more than 10,000 metres.

Almost rock-like in appearance, the 700 species of sea urchin can be found on the ocean floor or attached to coral or rock. The long, manoeuvring spines covering their bodies have nodules which enclose poison-secreting glands. On their underside can be found an apparatus called an Aristotle's lantern which also disperses poison. Stings from their tentacles are extremely painful resulting in cramp, shock and vomiting.

The sea snake is related to the land snake but has evolved an oar-like tail and flattened body. The majority of sea snakes can be found in coastal areas and estuaries of Asia and Australasia, although there is one species – recognized by its yellow underbelly – which can be found throughout the Pacific. Although slow to strike, the sea snake is venomous; a bite necessitates immediate attention to neutralize the poison.

Sea anemones and urchins have venom in their tentacles and spines which can become lodged in the skin, so extraction of these is painful but essential. The sea snake resorts to the traditional bite with fangs. Once the tentacles or spines have been removed, bathe the area in a disinfectant wash using the following formula, which could be prepared prior to your departure:

2 drops lavender oil
1 drop peppermint oil
1 drop tea tree oil
100 ml distilled water

Follow by applying five drops of neat lavender oil directly to the area of the sting or bite until emergency services arrive.

While you are recovering from the bite, drink plenty of warm fluid (at least two litres a day) and massage the whole body with the following formula:

1 drop eucalyptus oil
2 drops geranium oil
1 drop tea tree oil
20 ml base oil

Wrap up warm in bed and apply neat lavender oil (five drops) to the sting or bite as often as possible. In the case of sea urchins and stingrays (*see* FISH BITES), the discomfort can last for up to three days, so keep to this routine until you have recovered.

Sea Travel

When travelling by sea, especially for the first time, seasickness can make for a daunting and embarrassing experience. The rough movements of a yacht are vastly different to cruising on an ocean liner, yet passengers on both may succumb to reaching for starboard!

The feeling of imbalance experienced is due to your senses delivering conflicting messages to the brain. Fix your eyes upon the horizon or a stationary object. Place a drop or two of peppermint oil on a tissue or handkerchief and, if you feel an imminent convulsion, inhale deeply from it.

Skin Care

The skin is the largest organ of the body, comprising the epidermis (protective layer) and the dermis (deeper layer). It protects the internal organs from injury and bacterial invasion. Functioning as a heat regulator, the blood and sweat glands in the skin adjust to outside temperatures to maintain the internal temperature of a healthy body (37° Celsius/98° Fahrenheit). Sebaceous and sweat glands in the skin help the excretory process by removing excess moisture, toxins and fats from the body, which is constantly adjusting to internal and external influences. These influences are registered by the rich nerve supply present in the skin, responding to heat, cold, touch, pressure and pain. The skin has restricted powers of absorption: essential oils, fatty substances and drugs can be absorbed by the skin, whereas water and alcohol are not absorbed at all.

Dry Skin

Dry skin looks and feels taut, wrinkles easily and requires daily nourishing to prevent dehydration. Travelling to an unfamiliar climate can result in dry skin, not necessarily from endless sunbathing. Whether you are hiking in Yosemite, California or skiing in the Swiss Alps, your skin may be vulnerable to drying.

If your skin has a tendency to be dry, invest in regular body rubs prior to your travels with the following body oil formula, which is great for hydrating and nourishing the skin:

> 1 drop chamomile oil
> 2 drops geranium oil
> 1 drop lavender oil
> 20 ml base oil/cream

This rich skin oil should be used in small amounts on the face and body like a moisturizer but is not to be applied to the eye area. Use 2.5–5 ml on the face, massaging in an upward motion. Leave for a minute or so then blot the excess with a tissue. You can decant the mixture for day-trips or add the essential oils to your preferred vegetable-based moisturizing cream.

Pay attention to your diet. The old axiom 'you are what you eat' has particular relevance while travelling. Including plenty of fruit and vegetables in your diet will increase energy levels and boost the elasticity of your skin. Drink plenty of bottled water while away, but avoid large amounts of caffeine, as found in tea, coffee and cola drinks. Herbal teas are refreshing alternatives and an excellent way to cleanse your body gently and hydrate your skin cells. As 98 per cent of the body is made up of water, hydrating your skin is an external and internal affair.

Oily Skin

Travelling to a hot, sunny climate is a blessing to someone with an oily and/or blemished skin. The sun's rays release blocked pores, encourage

sebaceous flow and promote an even colour. To capitalize on this, replace astringents with floral waters,
such as the following formula, which can help to
balance oil flow and skin regeneration:

1 drop geranium oil
200 ml distilled water

The formula should always be shaken before use.
Saturate a cotton pad with the solution and wipe
across the face – or you may find a spray bottle more
handy.

No matter how oily your skin condition, nourishing the skin surface is important to maintain elasticity and suppleness. Add the following to your
preferred moisturizing cream (the best ones are
based on organic cold-pressed oils and contain no
petrochemicals), or you may mix the formula with
a base oil containing sesame, a natural sun filter:

2 drops geranium oil
1 drop lavender oil
1 drop rosemary oil
20 ml base oil/cream

Apply a small amount to your face and neck (avoiding the eye area), massaging in circular movements.
Leave the oil for a few minutes then blot off the
excess. For the occasional spot, apply neat lavender
oil daily until the blemish subsides; refrain from
picking spots as you will probably damage skin tis-

sue and increase the spread of infection under the skin.

Snakes

Snakes can be found in many different climates all around the world. There are, however, no indigenous snakes in New Zealand or Ireland. Not all snakes are poisonous. The ones you are most likely to encounter, or at least be aware of, on your travels are the snakes which fall under the categories of the elapids and the vipers.

Elapids

The elapids group consists of 220 species of venomous snakes, including the cobras and African mambas. They can usually be identified by their slim-to-medium build, although there are exceptions to the rule – large ones! They can be found in Africa, Asia, southern North America, Central and South America and some parts of Australasia. No elapids are found in Europe.

Their venom is so potent that even a scratch from a fang could be fatal. The characteristic fixed fangs sit in the upper jaw, and within their structure are venom canals which make delivery of poison convenient, to say the least. As well as poisoning their adversaries through biting, the cobra can spray venom from a distance of up to two metres covering an arc of half a metre in width to ensure splattering the intended victim.

Here is a guide to the elapids you are most likely to encounter (hopefully not!) when visiting a specified region:

Common cobra — various locations: urban localities, paddy fields, grassland

Egyptian cobra — usually dry locales such as savannahs; sometimes found near water

King cobra — rural, agricultural, forest areas

Black mamba — savannah, thickets, depleting forests, rocky terrain

Green mamba — forests, depleting forests, thickets

Elapid bites result in a temporary (sometimes fatal) attack on the central nervous system. Symptoms include irregular breathing and difficulty in swallowing or speaking.

Vipers

The 160 species of viper can be found in the more temperate climes of Europe, Asia and North America. Distinguished by their triangular heads, they are usually short but vary in build.

Vipers have a refined venom apparatus. Their folding fangs lie in the roof of the mouth when the jaws are closed. Rather than bite, vipers stab by striking at their intended victim at lightning speed; so rapid is the act, that a viper can strike and resume a defensive position within seconds. For your reference, here are some of the most common types:

European adder — heaths, moors, railway embankments, quarries

Gaboon viper — depleting forests, thickets, rainforests

Malayan pit viper — cultivated areas, forest

Saw scaled viper —   semi-desert, arid regions
Western diamond/ — some cultivated areas, semi-desert,
Back rattlesnake   arid areas

Viper bites manifest in a whole range of physical symptoms such as swelling of the limbs and abnormal bleeding from the injection sites, gums and skin. Bloodclotting can also occur.

Poisonous venom is life-threatening. Once bitten by a snake, remember the golden rule: do not remove the venom from the bitten area, no matter what you have seen in the movies! This act can disperse the venom quickly through the body. If the skin is punctured by two teeth marks, the bite is more than likely poisonous, coming from one of the groups above. Send or call for the emergency medical service immediately.

In the meantime, the following steps can buy you some valuable time. Wash the bitten area with any liquid to hand as you need to wash away as much venom as possible to decrease the amount absorbed. It is imperative that circulation to the affected area is restricted, so tie a bandage, bandanna, tie or handkerchief around the limb so it is comfortably secure, but not numbing in its effect.

Lavender tends to have a neutralizing effect on the venom of vipers. Apply five to eight drops of neat lavender essential oil to the affected area, depending on its size. Drip a few drops directly onto the skin, being careful not to tamper with the bitten locality.

You are more than likely to be detained for at least 12 hours in the intensive-care unit of the local hospital, where a doctor would immediately give a tetanus booster to counteract the poison. Only in cases of extreme poisoning of the system would the doctor administer antivenom, and that is usually several hours after the bite.

Spider Bites

These creepy-crawlies can present you with an unwanted keepsake: a nasty bite. Always check your shoes as spiders find them a cosy hiding place. If the worst happens, seek medical attention as soon as possible. Vigilance is called for when travelling to a tropical or subtropical climate, although venomous spiders are not unheard of in more temperate regions.

Black Widow

The black widow spider is usually found lurking under logs in fields and woodland. There are six known species, and it is the female that has the lethal reputation – more from her relations with the male of the species than the effect of her bite on humans (she mauls him to death after familiar relations!). Although venomous, the bite is rarely lethal to an adult. It does, however, cause severe pain and a mild paralysis of the diaphragm. This is usually accompanied by nausea and vomiting, depending upon the severity of poisoning.

Brown Recluse

This plain-looking spider deserves a reputation. Most commonly found in the western and southern United States, it favours dark corners and stones under which to hide. A bite is occasionally fatal, as the quick-acting venom destroys the walls of the blood vessels surrounding the pierce, resulting in a sizeable skin ulcer. Depending upon the victim's immunity, it can take several months to heal.

Immediately wash the affected area with the following antiseptic formula, which should be shaken before use. If there is none prepared, wash out the bite with whatever liquid you can find:

2 drops lavender oil
1 drop peppermint oil
1 drop tea tree oil
100 ml distilled water

Apply three to five drops of neat lavender oil to halt and neutralize the bite. Reapply as often as necessary once the essence has been absorbed by the skin, while waiting for emergency services.

Sprains

Wrong-footing can cause an excruciatingly painful sprain or a twisted ankle. Make a compress by soaking a small towel or flannel in ice-cold water, squeezing until semi-dry then applying to the sprained area to reduce swelling. Reapply as often as necessary to reduce discomfort. Follow up with a bandage-compress soaked in the following aromatic solution. The bandage should ideally be long enough to wrap around the swelling, secured with a pin and left overnight:

> 1 drop chamomile oil
> 1 drop eucalyptus oil
> 1 drop lavender oil
> 2.5 ml base oil
> 200 ml warm water

Once the bandage has been removed, apply three drops of neat lavender oil to the area daily to encourage the repair of damaged tissue. If the swelling does not subside after 24 hours, the injury could be fracture, so visit a doctor as soon as possible.

Sunburn

The sun makes us feel good so it is no wonder that we flock to sunny climes for our holidays or even to live. As human beings, we need the sun: its rays enable our bodies to manufacture vitamin D, essential for healthy growth and bones. Almost everyone notices a great improvement in skin texture and tone once it is exposed to the sun. Skin disorders such as acne and eczema heal quickly under its influence. The psychological benefits of sunlight are now widely recognized as well. It is thought that a lack of sunlight can contribute to depression, such as in the condition seasonal affective disorder (SAD), which affects some people during the winter.

For all the sun's benefits, however, there are dangers too. We now know that skin cancer is directly linked to sunbathing, and that this may be due to the depletion of the ozone layer which leaves us inadequately protected from the sun's harmful ultraviolet rays. Common sense coupled with adequate sun protection are the only tools we have to protect ourselves. Limit sunbathing to three hours a day, avoiding the period between noon and 3 p.m. when the sun is at its most powerful. Even if you tan easily and never burn, shield yourself from ultraviolet rays with a sunscreen of at least factor 10. Cover your head and hair with a hat or use the hair formula described on page 72. Protect your eyes by investing in a good pair of sunglasses.

After sunbathing, take a soothing, aromatic

chamomile bath, using the following formula:

4 drops chamomile oil
5 ml base oil

Follow by applying liberal amounts of the following after-sun oil. You should not use oil on the skin while sunbathing as this will make you 'fry', which could result in damaged skin.

1 drop chamomile oil
1 drop geranium oil
1 drop lavender oil
1 drop tea tree oil
20 ml base oil

Applying the after-sun oil regularly nourishes your skin, prolongs the tan, soothes sunburn and builds a resistance to future sunburn.

Cases of severe sunburn should be treated immediately by a doctor. In the meantime, apply a cold compress directly to the burn and surrounding area. Do not use oily substances to treat the burn. Lavender is the only oil that can be used neat, directly on the skin (*see* BURNS).

For cooling down while on the beach, refreshing yourself and your surroundings, spray yourself regularly with a fine mist of the following formula:

1 drop eucalyptus oil
2 drops lavender oil
1 drop peppermint oil
200 ml (spray bottle) distilled water

The formula should be shaken vigorously before use.

Sunstroke

Exposing yourself to the sun's rays for long periods when you are unaccustomed to the climate and heat intensity is asking for trouble. Not only will there be an increased risk of skin cancer through sunburn (*see page* 115), but you could also suffer from sunstroke.

Sunstroke creeps up on you: the drowsiness, headaches, dehydration, dry mouth and fluctuating body temperature are some of the reactions your body experiences before you eventually pass out. These are signals that the heat regulation system in your body is malfunctioning. The body temperature needs to be brought down and lost fluids replenished as soon as possible. The following treatment helps this process and should be continued for at least 48 hours until the body adjusts to normal temperature (37° Celsius/98° Fahrenheit):

1 drop chamomile oil
3 drops eucalyptus oil
2.5 ml base oil

Add the mixture to a lukewarm bath, swirling the water to disperse the essences, and sponge down the body. You should take two to three such baths per day over a 48-hour period for this treatment to be effective. Drink a minimum of two litres of water per day (adding a teaspoon of salt); on the third day decrease to a litre per day and, wherever possible for the duration of your trip, maintain this fluid intake.

Toothache

Whether it is a loose tooth, sensitive gums or a raw nerve keeping you up at night, essential oils can temporarily alleviate pain and discomfort until you can be seen by the local dentist. Peppermint essential oil acts as an analgesic when applied directly to the offending tooth, and is an excellent mouth purifier. This accounts for the widespread use of this antiviral essential oil in most toothpastes. Make a solution with:

> 1 drop peppermint oil
> 50 ml warm water

Swirl the water vigorously to disperse the essence. Soak a cotton bud in the solution and apply directly to the painful tooth and surrounding gum area.

A hot compress applied to the jawbone can reduce pain considerably. Use the following formula:

> 1 drop lavender oil
> 1 drop peppermint oil
> 5 ml base oil
> 500 ml hot water

A massage oil for the jawbone can be made by omitting the water, doubling the amount of base oil but using the same dosage of essential oils.

Upset Stomach

It is not uncommon to feel queasy or have an upset stomach while travelling (*see SEA TRAVEL*). Poorly prepared food or foods washed with contaminated water supplies can also cause a stomach upset. When visiting another country, experiencing different foods and water can play havoc with your digestive processes – unless you are blessed with a 'cast-iron stomach'. The first week or so is a period of adjustment which, in the worst scenario, can be accompanied by intermittent bouts of diarrhoea and constipation as the body cleanses itself of the offending substances.

Drinking plenty of bottled or distilled water can help this cleansing operation. Garlic capsules are also useful as the antibiotic properties neutralize harmful bacteria without hindering the function of friendly bacteria which maintain the equilibrium of the stomach. Two capsules a day are all that is needed to purify and strengthen the circulatory and lymphatic systems (*see GARLIC*).

Help is also at hand with the following massage oil, designed to alleviate discomfort and restore balance. Paying particular attention to the abdomen and the lower back area to stimulate the kidneys:

2 drops geranium oil
1 drop peppermint oil
1 drop rosemary oil
20 ml base oil

Continue drinking plenty of water throughout your trip.

Wasps
(*see* BEES)

Quick-reference Chart

Use this chart to see, at a glance, which essential oils can be used for a variety of common ailments. It also tells you the ways in which the oils can be used. Do not use this chart until you are familiar with guidelines for using essential oils safely. For further information, turn to the relevant page in Chapter 3, the *A-Z of Ailments and Aromatherapy Treatments*.

	Bath	Compress	Massage Oil
Aches	Lavender 2 Rosemary 3 Base 2.5 ml		Eucalyptus 1 Rosemary 1 Lavender 2 Base 20 ml
Air travel	Geranium 3 Lavender 2 Base 2.5 ml		Chamomile 1 Geranium 2 Lavender 1 Base 20 ml
Anxiety	(for children) Lavender 1 Chamomile 1 or Geranium 1 Base 2.5 ml (for adults) Chamomile 2 Lavender 2 Base 2.5 ml		
Arrival			
Atmosphere			

Spray/Wash	Vapour Ring	Tissue/ Handkerchief	Neat Application
	Lavender 5		
Lavender 1			
5 drops total from any combination of the following: Geranium 5 Lavender 5 Lemongrass Rosemary Tea tree			

	Bath	**Compress**	**Massage Oil**
Backache	Eucalyptus 2		Chamomile 2
	Peppermint 1		Rosemary 1
	Rosemary 1		Base 10 ml
	Base 5 ml		
Backpacking	Eucalyptus 3		Eucalyptus 1
	Lavender 1		Lemongrass 2
	Tea tree 1		Peppermint 1
	Base 2.5 ml		Base 20 ml
Bruises		Chamomile 1	
		Lavender 1	
		Base 10 ml	
Bees			
Burns			
Camping	Eucalyptus 2		Eucalyptus
	Lavender 1		Lemongrass
	Tea tree 1		Peppermint
	Base 2.5 ml		Sesame oil
			20 ml
Chapped lips			Chamomile 1
			Lavender 1
			Base 10 ml
Colds	Eucalyptus 3		Eucalyptus 1
	Geranium 2		Rosemary 1
	Base 2.5 ml		Base 10 ml

Spray/Wash	Vapour Ring	Tissue/ Handkerchief	Neat Application
Eucalyptus 1 Lavender 2 Tea tree 1 Warm water 100 ml			Lavender 3–5 Lemon juice 1 tsp
	Eucalyptus 1 Lemongrass 3 Peppermint 1		
		Eucalyptus 2	

	Bath	Compress	Massage Oil
Constipation			Rosemary 1 Peppermint 1 Base 10 ml
Cramp			Eucalyptus 1 Geranium 1 Base 10 ml
Cuts			
Dry skin			Chamomile 1 Geranium 2 Lavender 1 Base oil/cream 20 ml
Dysentery	Eucalyptus 1 Tea tree 1 Lavender 2 Base 5 ml		Eucalyptus 1 Tea tree 1 Lavender 2 Base 20 ml
Fainting			
Feet			Eucalyptus 1 Lavender 1 Base 10 ml
Fever	Chamomile 1 Eucalyptus 1 Lemongrass 2 Base 2.5 ml	Eucalyptus 1 Lemongrass 1 Base 5 ml	
Fish bites			

Spray/Wash	Vapour Ring	Tissue/ Handkerchief	Neat Application
Lavender 2 Tea tree 1 Base 2.5 ml			Lavender 5
Geranium 1			
Eucalyptus 1 Tea tree 1 Lavender 2 Distilled water 100 ml		Peppermint 2 or Rosemary 2	
	Lavender 4 Tea tree 1		Lavender 5
Lavender 2 Peppermint 1 Tea tree 1 Base 2.5 ml			

	Bath	Compress	Massage Oil
Frostbite			Eucalyptus 1 Geranium 2 Rosemary 1 Base 20 ml
Hair protector			Rosemary 2 Chamomile 1 Lavender 1 Base 20 ml
Hair (oily)			Rosemary 3 Geranium 5 Eucalyptus 1 Shampoo/ conditioner 100 ml
Hair (dry)			Rosemary 5 Chamomile 2 Lavender 2 Shampoo/ conditioner 100 ml
Hayfever			Chamomile 1 Lemongrass 1 Tea tree 1 Base 15 ml
Headache	Lavender 3 Rosemary 2 Base 2.5 ml		Lavender 1 Peppermint 1 Base 10 ml
Indigestion			Peppermint 1 Rosemary 1 Base 10 ml

Spray/Wash	Vapour Ring	Tissue/Handkerchief	Neat Application
Chamomile 1 or Rosemary 1			
Chamomile 1 or Rosemary 1			
		Chamomile 1 Lemongrass 1	
			Lavender 2

	Bath	**Compress**	**Massage Oil**
Insect bites			
Insect-repellent	Eucalyptus 1 Lemongrass 2 Peppermint 1 Base 20 ml		
Insomnia	Chamomile 1 Lavender 3 Base 2.5 ml		
Jet-lag	Geranium 1 Lavender 2 Lemongrass 1 Base 2.5 ml		Geranium 2 Lavender 2 Base 20 ml
	Chamomile 1 Geranium 1 Lavender 1 Base 2.5 ml		
	Eucalyptus 2 Geranium 1 Rosemary 3 Base 2.5 ml		
Mouthwash			

Spray/Wash	Vapour Ring	Tissue/Handkerchief	Neat Application
Eucalyptus 1 Lavender 2 Tea tree 1 Warm water 100 ml			Lavender 5
Eucalyptus 1 Lemongrass 3 Peppermint 1 Tea tree 1 Distilled water 100 ml	Lavender 2 Lemongrass 3		
Peppermint 1 or Rosemary 1 Distilled water 200 ml			

	Bath	Compress	Massage Oil
Mosquito bites			
Muscular pain			Eucalyptus 1 Lavender 1 Rosemary 2 Base 20 ml
Nettle rash			Chamomile 1 Tea tree 1 Base 10 ml
Nosebleeds			
Oily skin			Geranium 2 Lavender 1 Rosemary 1 Base oil/cream 20 ml
Premenstrual tension	Geranium 3 Lavender 1 Rosemary 2 Base 2.5 ml		Geranium 2 Rosemary 2 Base 20 ml
Prickly heat	Eucalyptus 2 Lavender 1 Base 2.5 ml		

Spray/Wash	Vapour Ring	Tissue/ Handkerchief	Neat Application
Eucalyptus 1 Lemongrass 2 Tea tree 1 Distilled water 100 ml			Lavender 5
			Lavender 3–5
		Lavender 2	
Geranium 1 Distilled water 200ml			
		Geranium 1	
Lavender 1 Peppermint 1 Base 5ml Distilled water 500 ml			

	Bath	Compress	Massage Oil
Sea creatures			Eucalyptus 1 Geranium 2 Tea tree 1 Base 20 ml
Sea travel			
Snake bites			
Spider bites			
Sprains			
Sunburn	Chamomile 4 Base 5 ml		Chamomile 1 Geranium 1 Lavender 1 Tea tree 1 Base 20 ml
Sunstroke	Eucalyptus 3 Chamomile 1 Base 2.5 ml		
Toothache		Lavender 1 Peppermint 1	Lavender 1 Peppermint 1 Base oil 10 ml
Upset stomach			Geranium 2 Peppermint 1 Rosemary 1 Base oil 20 ml

Spray/Wash	Vapour Ring	Tissue/ Handkerchief	Neat Application
Lavender 2 Peppermint 1 Tea tree 1 Distilled water 100 ml			Lavender 5
		Peppermint 2	
			Lavender 5–8
			Lavender 3–5
Eucalyptus 1 Lavender 2 Peppermint 1 Distilled water 200 ml			

Immunization – Useful Information

Immunization is essential when travelling to certain countries, and advisable for most other destinations. Contracting malaria or typhoid in southern Europe is just as much of a risk as in more tropical climates.

You should begin a course of immunization treatments at a suitable time before your departure date, allowing for adequate spacing of doses. Your doctor will be able to advise you on your requirements. Apart from the 'modern' vaccinations available from your doctor, there are also effective alternative treatments in the form of homoeopathy. *A Handbook of Homoeopathic Alternatives to Immunisation* by Susan Curtis (Winter Press, available from Neals Yard Remedies) is a practical guide to the medications available. (You should be aware that peppermint essential oil can act as an antidote to some homoeopathic medications.)

Cholera

Cholera can be contracted from contaminated food and water in areas where there is poor sanitation, such as in parts of Africa, Asia, South America and the Middle East. Although the World Health Organization has ruled that certification of immunization is no longer required by any country or region, some countries do request documents from travellers entering from high-risk areas. One immunization dose is required for certification, which is valid after six days for six months. The vaccine is not to be given to children under six months.

Hepatitis A

A virus spread by the faeces, hepatitis is endemic worldwide. Vaccine is usually offered at the same time as the typhoid immunization, as exposure to one infection increases the risk of exposure to the other. The well-seasoned tropical traveller may well have the antibodies present to be immune to this symptomatic infection. However, if the antibodies are not present (the test is widely available), the vaccine should be given just before departure and repeated every six months. When returning from an area where hepititis is prevalent, it is advisable to boost the vaccine to prevent secondary infections of the liver.

Malaria

A resurgence of the malaria virus has occurred since the 1960s in parts of South America, the Indian sub-continent and even Turkey. As yet, there is no totally effective vaccine. Prophylactic tablets are prescribed to those likely to be exposed to the most life-threatening form of mosquito which can be found in Africa and Asia. The tablets should be taken at least one week before your trip to gain the necessary level of tolerance in the blood, thereby reducing the risk of infection. These tablets are not curative once infection has taken place, so regular doses are essential for effectiveness during your travels as well as for four weeks after your return.

Tetanus

Tetanus vaccine is recommended for all individuals, travelling or not. The infection is caused by a virus found in soil. The illness affects the spinal cord, manifesting as spasms, firstly in the jaw (lockjaw). After your first dose of three vaccines, a booster is required every 10 years.

Typhoid

Typhoid fever is endemic worldwide. Transmitted via the faeces, it is a reflection of poor hygiene and living standards. Immunization is not necessary for destinations with public health standards, such as Europe, North America, Australasia and Japan. Injections or medication is recommended, however, when travelling to high-risk areas, especially if the travelling itinerary is overland or adventure-oriented. The vaccine from the doctor comprises two doses separated by four to six weeks, and provides immunity for three years.

Yellow Fever

This disease is caused by a virus which infects monkeys in tropical forested areas. It may be transmitted to humans by mosquitoes who usually prey on the monkeys. Immunization protects the individual and prevents the spread of the disease to urban developments. A single vaccination is effective for 10 years and, as in the case of cholera immunization, a certificate is provided which the traveller may be requested to produce when travelling from a high-risk area. This vaccine is not suitable for pregnant women or babies under nine months old.

Seeking Help

If the unfortunate occurs during your travels and you have to seek urgent medical attention, you may experience difficulty in communicating your needs unless you are fluent in the local language. The International Association for Medical Assistance for Travellers issues directories which list doctors that speak English, French, German or Japanese. Membership is free, but the organization welcomes voluntary donations for the service it provides. This Association also has useful information on climates, acclimatization and immunization. For further details, write to the International Association for Medical Assistance to Travellers, Gotthardstrasse 17, CH–6300 Zug, Switzerland.

Travel Information

Airlines

The airlines listed below have taken a unique approach to service in the skies or on the ground. Contact the airline in your locality for details of services and flight reservations.

AIR NEW ZEALAND
Winner of the Business Traveller's Best Airline to South Pacific Award for nine years running, Air New Zealand is renowned for its amicable service. The airline offers a best-selling 'Revival on Arrival' aromatherapy kit, via the in-flight magazine. As the name implies, the kit is designed to refresh the senses upon arrival. It has been formulated by London-based aromatherapist Danièle Ryman.

BRITISH AIRWAYS
Providing a unique and friendly service, British Airways operate travel clinics all over the UK dealing with enquiries ranging from immunization to visas. Two walk-in centres are available in London for all travellers:

156 Regent Street
London W1R 5TA

Gatwick London Terminal
Victoria Place
115 Buckingham Palace Road
London SW1W 9SJ

JAPAN AIR

Japan Air has recently started to offer three types of shiatsu massage to passengers travelling first-class. Regular customers greeted the service with 'enthusiasm and surprise'. Shiatsu is an ancient form of Japanese massage, which involves stimulating and relaxing the body's energy points (known as *tsubos*) along the Yin and Yang energy meridians of the body. Immediate benefits include increased relaxation, lowered blood pressure and an energy boost, depending upon which of the three types of treatment you choose.

VIRGIN ATLANTIC

The first airline to introduce in-flight massage using essential oils to business-class passengers. The success of this service has prompted Virgin to open the first pre-flight treatment centre in London's Heathrow airport, within the Upper Class lounge. A manicure is also part of the service.

Insurance

It is strongly recommended that you take out appropriate travel insurance before setting off on your trip. All the airlines and travel companies listed in this appendix offer their own form of insurance. Some companies specialize in, for example, adventure or trekking holidays.

Travel Companies

UK

EXODUS
Head office
9 Weir Road
London SW12 OLT
(0181) 673 0859

Specializing in overland, adventure and active cultural explorations in all continents, Exodus has 20 years' experience in satisfying the traveller's wanderlust. All the tours are hosted by local guides, and accommodation is provided by excellent small, family-run guesthouses or lodges. The company prides itself on its work with governments of destination countries in preserving the environment.

RIVER ISLAND EXPEDITIONS
West World
West Gate
London W5 1XP
(0181) 810 4525

This travel company provides a unique travel service via the company's retail clothing operation across the UK. Apart from adventure holidays and short breaks – including ballooning weekends, rafting down the Zambezi and participating in a Wyoming cattle drive – the company has an informative Discovery membership club which entitles members to discounts on 47 adventures across the globe, and a chance to enter into prize draws.

TRIPS
24 Clifton Wood Crescent
Clifton Wood
Bristol BS8 4TU
(0117) 9292 199

The first choice for those with a special interest in Belize, Mexico and the rest of Central America, Trips can either book your flight or design a fully inclusive holiday to suit your budget, especially if your area of interest includes archaeology or diving. Advocating 'sustainable tourism', Trips consults with conservation groups and local guides to ensure monies spent help support local communities and environmental projects.

Australia

EXODUS
Suite 5, Level 5
95–99 York Street
Sydney
New South Wales 2000
(02) 299 6355

Belgium

JOKER TOERISME/TOURISM
Boondaalsesteenweg 6
Chaussee de Boondael 6
1050 Bruxelles
(02) 648 78 78

Canada

G.A.P
227 Sterling Road
Suite 105
Toronto
Ontario M6R 2B2
(416) 535 6600

Denmark

TOPAZ GLOBETROTTERKLUB
Bakkeleyvej 2
8680 Ry
86 89 36 22

Germany

EXPLORER
Huttenstrasse 17
40215 Dusseldorf
(0211) 99 49 02

Greece

TROPICAL TOURS
11 Voukourestiou St
Athens 106 71
(01) 360 7168

Netherlands

TERRA TRAVEL
Haarlemmerstraat 24–26
1013 ER Amsterdam
(020) 627 5129

New Zealand

ADVENTURE WORLD
101 Great South Road
PO Box 74
008 Remuera
Auckland
524 5118

Portugal

SITTIS
Calcada Ribeiro Santos 3
1200 Lisboa
(01) 397 10 07

South Africa

KUONI TRAVEL
4th Floor
94 President Street
Johannesburg 2001
11 297 434

Spain

GROUP ITSASLUR
C/ Goroabe 25, Bajo
31005 Pamplona
Navarra
(948) 24 27 91

Switzerland

EXODUS
Rain 35
POB 2226
5001 Aarau
(064) 22 76 63

USA

SAFARI CENTRE
3201 North Sepulveda Boulevard
Manhattan Beach
California CA 90266
(310) 546 4411

Spas and Retreats

Another type of appealing holiday is one spent relaxing, being totally pampered at a health spa or secluded vacation retreat. Here, you can enjoy various body therapies, such as aromatherapy or shiatsu, or participate in relaxation and stress-management workshops which can be put into practice once back at home.

USA

HEALTH TREK
115 South Topanga Canyon Boulevard
Ste. 185 Topanga
California 90290
(310) 4155 4204

Specialists in health resorts, spas and retreats to suit your budget and your lifestyle. Destinations include California and Denver in the USA, the Bahamas, Mexico, Sweden, Switzerland and Japan.

AVEDA

Aveda Spa Osceola
1015 Cascade Street
Route 3, box 72
Osceola
Wisconsin 540 20
(715) 294 4465

West Indies (Dominican Republic)

LA MANSION CONCIERGE OFFICE

126 East 56th Street
New York
New York 10022
(800) 826 1550

Retailers and Suppliers

A good selection of essential oils and aromatherapy-based travel products can be found in your local health-food store as well as from the following suppliers.

AVEDA ESTHETIQUE
An American company with outlets worldwide, Aveda supplies aromatherapy-based beauty products, many of which come in handy travel sizes. You can also buy vapour rings and travel pouches for essential oils. Mail-order service available.

Harvey Nichols
109 Knightsbridge
London SW1 7RJ

Liberty
Regent Street
London W1R 6AH

Australia

Shop 318 (Little Collins Street Entrance)
Collins Street
Melbourne 3000

Shop 303 Melbourne Central
Lonsdale Street
Melbourne 3000

Singapore

Takashimaya Shopping Centre
391 Orchard Road
B1–54
Ngee Ann City
Singapore 0923

USA

8500 Beverly Boulevard 601
Los Angeles
California CA 90048

400 Central Avenue Southeast
Minneapolis
Minnesota MN 55408

509 Madison Avenue
New York NY 10022

8047L Tysons Corner Centre
McLean
Virginia VA 22102

1075 Bellevue Square
Bellevue
Washington WA 98004

1015 Cascade Street
Route 3, Box 72
Osceola
Wisconsin WI 54020

THE BODY SHOP
The Body Shop has over 100 shops in the UK and a further 170 outlets in the USA. You will also find this store throughout Europe, and there are branches opening in the Far East and Australasia. With such a prominence across the globe, the company has established itself as a leader in the cosmetic industry with an environmentally concerned ethos. Products include travel-size hair and skin-care products utilizing essential oils and herbs. Also available are travel accessories and an extensive suncare range. For the branch nearest to you, consult the telephone directory or contact the following address:

THE BODY SHOP INTERNATIONAL
Hawthorn Road
Wick
Little Hampton
West Sussex

CULPEPER

Products include essential oils, travel bags and boxes and eye compresses. Mail-order service available. Consult your local telephone directory for your nearest branch.

UK

8 The Market
Covent Garden
London WC2E 8RB
7 New Inn Hall Street
Oxford
OX1 2DH

Japan

K F Bldg
3–Chome 6
Kita Aoyama
Munatu
Tokyo 10

JURILIQUE

This Australian company supplies essential oils, travel-size skincare, travel containers, vapour rings and travel pouches. It also distributes to various health-food outlets. Contact the numbers below for your nearest store.

Australia

Austral Biolab Pty. Ltd.,
PO Box 522
Mount Barker
South Australia 5251

UK

Unit 11, Chelsea Wharf
15 Lots Road
London SW10 0QJ

NEALS YARD

Products available from this British company include essential oils, base oils, herbs, travel bags, travel-size soaps, travel bottles and atomizers, suncare and books. Mail order service available.

UK

15 Neals Yard
Covent Garden
London WC2H 9DP

Chelsea Farmers Market
Sydney Street
Chelsea
London SW1 6NR

5 Golden Cross
Cornmarket Street
Oxford OX1 3EU

Australia

Remo
Oxford Street
(At Crown Street)
Sydney 2010

USA

The distributor listed below can refer you to your nearest outlet. Cities with outlets include Los Angeles, Houston and New York.

2415 3rd Street
Suite 240
San Francisco
California CA 94107

Professional Associations

HOSPITAL FOR TROPICAL DISEASES TRAVEL CLINIC HELPLINE

For up-to-date information on what protection is needed where, call (0839) 337733.

INTERNATIONAL ASSOCIATION FOR MEDICAL ASSISTANCE TO TRAVELLERS

Gotthardstrasse 17
CH–6300 Zug
Switzerland

INTERNATIONAL FEDERATION OF AROMATHERAPISTS

Royal Masonic Hospital
Ravenscourt Park
London W6 0TN

INDEPENDENT PROFESSIONAL THERAPISTS INTERNATIONAL

Woodend
8 Ordsall Road
Retford
Notts. DN22 7PL

Glossary

Anatomy
The science of the structure and functions of the body.

Chlorofluorocarbons (CFCs)
Stable, non-toxic compound of fluorine and chlorine used as a propellant in aerosol cans, in the manufacture foam boxes for takeaway foods and as a refrigerant in refrigerators. Once released into the atmosphere they take, on average, seven years to reach the stratosphere where, under the influence of the sun's ultraviolet light, they destroy the chlorine atoms in the ozone layer which protects us from solar ultraviolet radiation.

Circulatory system
The movement of blood around the body. Oxygenated blood is carried from the heart through the arteries and capillaries to the tissues, returning waste matter to the heart through the veins.

Ecology
The study of the relationship of plants and animals (including humans!) to their environment and each other.

Endocrine system
Comprises glands that secrete hormones, the 'chemical messengers' that control all bodily functions.

Immune system
The body's system for fighting infection. Important elements are antibodies (produced by the spleen), lymph and white blood cells.

Keratin
The main constituent of hair, this protein is also found in skin.

Lymphatic system
A secondary circulatory system, lymph is the blood's waste-disposal outlet. It cleanses and drains toxic substances from the blood and is the first port of call for waste matter eliminated from the body via the skin and excretory systems (urine and faeces). Aromatherapy massage, exercise and a wholesome diet encourage healthy circulation of lymph around the body.

Molecules
All living things and inanimate objects are comprised of molecules. A molecule is the smallest unit into which a substance can be divided while maintaining the chemical components of that substance with at least two colliding atoms – the basis of matter.

Nervous system
The nerve cells of the body comprising neurones (the cell in the nerve that transmits electrical impulses), the nerves (congregations of fibres that take impulses from one part of the body to another), the spinal cord and the brain.

Stress
A natural human reaction – physical, mental or emotional – to external or internal influences. Without it, life would be very dull indeed. Stress can be a great motivator, but when handled incorrectly can result in panic attacks, anxiety, insomnia and even breathing difficulties. The pressures of modern living – demanding workloads, not being aware of one's limitations, high expectations and keeping up with the Joneses – have led to an increase in stress-related health problems. More important than the nature of the stressful event, however, is how a person reacts to and deals with it.

Synthetic
An artificially derived and manufactured substance.

Further Reading

Arcier M. *Aromatherapy*, Hamlyn (1990)

Baerheim A. & Svendsen J. *Essential Oils and Aromatic Plants*, International Symposium on Essential Oils, Nijhoff/Junk Publishers (Netherlands) (1985)

Culpeper, Nicholas. *The Complete Herbal*, Foulsham (1952)

Curtis, S. *A Handbook of Homeopathic Alternatives to Immunisation*, Winter Press (1994)

Curtis, S. & Fraser, R. *Natural Healing For Women*, Pandora (1991)

Davis, P. *Aromatherapy: An A–Z*, C.W. Daniel (1988)

Gattefossé, R.M. *Gattefossé's Aromatherapy* (ed. R. Tisserand), C.W. Daniel (1993)

Maury, M. *Marguerite Maury's Guide to Aromatherapy*, C.W. Daniel (1989)

Price, S. *Practical Aromatherapy*, Thorsons (1983)

Ryman, D. *The Aromatherapy Handbook*, C.W. Daniel (1988)

Simons, P. *Garlic*, Thorsons (1986)

Tisserand, M. *Aromatherapy for Women*, Thorsons (1985)

• Further Reading •

Valnet, J. *The Practice of Aromatherapy*, C.W. Daniel
   (1982)
Van Toller, S. & Dodd, G.H. *Fragrance — the Psychology
   and Biology of Perfume*, Elsevier Science Publishers
   (1992)
Worwood, V.A. *Aromantics*, Pan (1987)

Index